to the stutterer

speech foundation of america
publication no. 9

FIRST PRINTING — 1972
SECOND PRINTING — 1973
THIRD PRINTING — 1983
FOURTH PRINTING — 1988
FIFTH PRINTING — 1990

Published by
Speech Foundation of America
P.O. Box 11749
Memphis, Tennessee 38111

Library of Congress Catalog Card Number 76-376781
ISBN 0-933388-07-1

NOT COPYRIGHTED

This is a remarkable book of therapy advice. Nothing like it has ever been published before. What makes it unique and unusual is that every article in this book has been written by men and women who have been stutterers themselves. Each one of them has been 'through the mill' and knows what it is to have experienced the fear, anxiety and despair which is so often the lot of the stutterer. They know your problem.

Also all of the authors of these articles are now or have been speech pathologists. This means that they are experienced and trained in helping others with their speech problems—and they have written these articles to help you eliminate your stuttering. On the next three pages we list their twenty four names.

They represent a most distinguished array of authority and prestige in the field of stuttering. Included among them are sixteen who are or have been university professors of speech pathology, six who are or have been heads of speech pathology departments in such institutions, twelve who are or have been directors of speech and hearing clinics, and they include two psychiatrists, nine Fellows of the American Speech and Hearing Association and nine authors of books on the therapy of stuttering.

Although these writers do not all agree as to exactly what you should do to overcome your difficulty, there is a lot of uniformity in their recommendations and in their thinking. We believe that their ideas will help you. We are publishing this book in your interest and hope that you will make use of it.

Malcolm Fraser
Speech Foundation of America
June 1988

contents

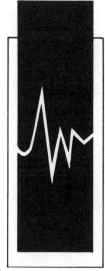

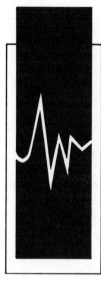

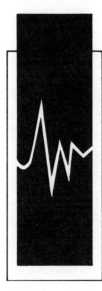

Express Yourself Or Go By Freight

Lon L. Emerick

One score and seven years ago, in a desperate attempt to cure their son's chronic speech problem, my parents spent their meagre savings to send me to a commercial school for stammering. Alas, to their dismay and my deepening feeling of hopelessness, it was just another futile attempt. While I rode woefully toward home on the train, a kindly old gray-haired conductor stopped at my seat and asked my destination. I opened my mouth for the well-rehearsed "Detroit" but all that emerged was a series of muted gurgles; I pulled my abdominal muscles in hard to break the terrifying constriction in my throat—silence. Finally, the old man peered at me through his bifocals, shook his head and, with just the trace of a smile, said, "Well, young man, either express yourself or go by freight."

The conductor had shuffled on down the aisle of the rocking passenger car before the shock waves swept over me. Looking out the window at the speeding landscape through a tearful mist of anger and frustration, I felt the surreptitious glances of passengers seated nearby; a flush of crimson embarrassment crept slowly up my neck and my head throbbed with despair. Long afterwards I remembered the conductor's penetrating comment. For years I licked that and other stuttering wounds and nursed my wrath to keep it warm, dreaming that someday I would right all those unrightable wrongs. But in the end his pithy pun changed my life. The old man, incredibly, had been right.

Why indeed go by freight? Why carry excess baggage, endure endless delays, languish forgotten and rejected in sooty siding yards, be bombarded with countless jolts and unplanned stops? Why let your journey through life be dictated by the time table of stuttering? Perhaps you too are searching for some way out of a morass of jumbled box cars and the maze of tracks that seem to lead only to empty, deadened spurs. Although it is difficult to give advice without seeing you and identifying your particular situation, I do know there are several things that have helped me and many other stutterers. May I extend this challenge to you: I invite you to do something difficult but with a sweet reward—to change the way you talk. The pathway to better speech is fraught with blind alleys, dark frightening tunnels and arduous climbs. Beware of any treatment that plumes itself in novelty and promises no pain; deep inside you know this cannot work. May I show you the trail?

The first thing you must do is admit to yourself that you need to change, that you really want to do something about the way you presently talk. This is tough but your commitment must be total; not even a small part of you must hold back. Don't dwell longingly on your fluency in the magical belief that someday your speech blocks will disappear. There is no magic potion, no pink pill that will cure stuttering. Don't sit around waiting for the right time, for an inspiration to come to you— *you must go to "it."* You must see that the old solutions, the things you have done to help yourself over the years (and those cover-up suggestions from well-meaning amateur therapists, "Think what you want to say," "Slow down," etc.) simply do not work. Ruts wear deep, though, and you will find it difficult to change; even though the way you presently talk is not particularly pleasant, it is familiar. It is the unknown from which we shrink.

You must be willing to endure temporary discomfort, perhaps even agony, for long range improvement. No one, except perhaps the quack, and there are still a few around, is promising you a rose garden. Why not take the time and effort now for a lifetime of freedom from your tangled tongue? How can you do that? You break down the global problem of stuttering into its smaller parts and then solve them one at a time. It's *simple*. No one said it was *easy*. Shall we begin?

1. Are you acquainted with your stuttering pattern? What do you *do* when you stutter? What can you *see, hear* and *feel*? Where are the triggers for those sticky blocks or runaway repetitions? How does your moment of stuttering progress from the first expectation you are going to stutter until the word is uttered? How do you release a block . . . an extra surge of energy, a sudden jerk of your head? I am asking you to observe closely what you do when you stutter; you can use a mirror, a tape recorder, your finger tips to search for areas of tension. A friend or relative whom you trust can also help you make a careful inventory. Stuttering is not some mysterious beast that

takes over your mouth—even though it may appear that way because it seems to occur so automatically. Stuttering is a series of activities that you *do*. It is your way of talking for now. Before you can change what you do, obviously you have to spend some time cataloging precisely what it is you do. Here is how one stutterer described his stuttering pattern:

> Can tell when I'm going to stutter . . . at least three words ahead. Tense my lower jaw. Purse my lips tightly . . . even when trying to say the /k/ sound! Blink my eyes shut and turn my head down and toward the right. I push harder and finally utter the word, "kite," by jerking my jaw forward.

2. Now, when you have a good idea of what you do when you stutter, set up a program of change. Take all the elements —the excess baggage—that make up your stuttering pattern and consciously and deliberately attempt to *add* (exaggerate), *vary* (instead of jerking your head to the right, jerk it to the left) and *drop* (stutter without that one mannerism) the separate aspects, one at a time. Start in an easy situation—alone, perhaps—and gradually increase the difficulty. Here is a chart that will help you organize your practice time:

head jerk	*Add*	*Vary*	*Drop*
	Monday, read aloud for 15 minutes.	Wednesday, read aloud for 15 minutes.	Friday, read aloud for 15 minutes.
	Exaggerate head jerk to the *left*.	*Exaggerate* easy head jerks to the *right*.	*Stop* use of head jerk.

(Follow this same plan for changing the other elements of your stuttering pattern; lip tensing, eye blink, etc.)

But, you say, I want to *stop* stuttering. Sure! But first you need to break up the habit pattern that you have built up over the years and this cannot be done instantly. The habit is powerful, because at the end of all the tension and struggle, the word does usually emerge. In a sense, then, stuttering works—so you persist in using the rituals that allow you to escape from stuttering. To break up a habit, you must alter its stereotyped nature.

3. When you are familiar with the various elements comprising your stuttering pattern and can alter them, then try to stutter more *easily* and *openly*. In a very real sense, the best

advice I can give you is that you must learn to stutter better, with a minimum of tension and hurry. Instead of pushing so hard, try to ease out of your blocks by sliding into the first syllable of the word; start the *movement* and *sound* flow at the same time and glide into the word. Use strong movements of your lips and jaw and *feel* the shifts in those structures as you move *forward* through a word. Much of the agony and consequent social punishment of stuttering comes from tensing and. holding back. Here are some instructions we gave to a stutterer recently who was learning to turn his stuttering on and off:

> When I raise my finger, you increase the pressure —to a real hard block. Then, as I lower my finger, slowly let the tension come out. That's right. Now, go back and forth on your own: increase and decrease the tension. Learn to play with your blocks this way; get the *feel* of coming out of those hard fixations.

4. Now I am going to ask you to do a strange thing: *to stutter on purpose.* I know, it sounds weird but it works. Why? Because it helps to drain away the fear (what have you got to hide if you are willing to stutter on purpose?) and it provides a lot of experience practicing the act of stuttering in a highly voluntary and purposeful manner. The more you stutter on purpose, the less you hold back; and the less you hold back, the less you stutter. We once worked with a young exchange student who almost completely extinguished her stuttering in one week by doing negative practice. We were enmeshed in doctoral examinations so we gave her a hand-counter and told her: "There are 100,000 people living in Lansing; see how many you can talk to and. show your stuttering." When I saw her seven days later she was haggard and worn but grinning broadly and not stuttering. Having taken us literally she had worked around the clock. Incredibly she had confronted 947 listeners! And she was totally unable to stutter involuntarily.

5. You must sharply reduce or eliminate the avoidances you use. Everytime you substitute one word for another, use a sound or some trick to get speech started, postpone or give up an attempt at talking, you make it harder for yourself. Instead of diminishing when evaded, fears incubate and grow. The avoider must maintain constant vigilance and continually devise new ways to elude the dreaded words, listeners or situations. It's like

pouring water into a leaking cask. Make a list of all your avoidances: What types do you use (starters, delaying tactics, etc.)? When, in what contexts do you use them? How frequently do you resort to evasion? In other words, prepare an avoidance inventory. Then, systematically vary and exaggerate each one; use the avoidances when you don't need to in a highly voluntary manner. Finally, when you find yourself using an avoidance involuntarily, invoke a self-penalty; for example, if you avoid the word "chocolate," you must then use that word several times immediately thereafter. One of the best penalties is to explain to the listener the avoidance you have just used and why you should resist such evasions.

6. No stutterer is an island. Peoples' reactions to you and your interpretations of their reactions have, as you know, a profound effect upon your speech. You need to go out and renew your acquaintance with listeners; you need to talk to all kinds of people in all kinds of situations. Set up daily quotas or challenges for yourself; enter those tough speaking situations and demonstrate to yourself that you can, even though stuttering, get the message across. Any adventure is more fun when shared with congenial and helpful companions. Fortunately, there is a group, the Council of Adult Stutterers with chapters in many parts of the country, that can provide information and support especially in this important aspect of altering old attitudes about your speech problem.

7. Strange as it seems, you may find it difficult to adjust to more fluent speech. For years you have been laboring from block to block, you have been speaking a stuttering language. And, if you have used stuttering as an excuse or crutch, you may feel naked and exposed without it. The best antidote is to practice your new fluency until it becomes familiar to you. Plug your ears and read aloud, feeling the flow of words; shadow-talk along with speakers on radio or television; enroll for a speech course in your local area.

Licking the problem of stuttering, mastering your own mouth, takes time; it cannot be accomplished overnight. How long it will take you I cannot say, for no two stutterers approach the challenge in the same way or move at the same rate but all have in common a beckoning mirage luring them ahead. Here then are the foundation blocks. Can you create from them stepping stones? Don't go any farther by freight. Express yourself!

Stuttering: What You Can Do About It

Margaret Rainey

I deeply wish that I could reach every stutterer in the world to tell the story I am about to tell here. Last evening, as a speech clinician, I gave a speech to a large group of people who were vitally interested in stutterers and in the nature of stuttering. This morning as I sit drinking my coffee, and while the memories and experiences of last evening are vivid, I want to share my feelings and my knowledge with as many stutterers as possible.

It is interesting that I had no fear of that audience. I had no dread of the monsters of fear that once reared their ugly heads and choked off my words and even my thoughts. Yes, I am a stutterer, and I hope that it will help any stutterer who may read this to know that I was such a severe stutterer that I could not put two meaningful words together until I was twenty-four years old. Do I still stutter? Oh, I call myself a stutterer because I still have small interruptions in my speech now and then. But there's another more important reason why I call myself a stutterer. *I'm not trying to hide the fact anymore!* I learned long ago that the harder I tried to camouflage my stuttering, the more severely I stuttered. It was a vicious circle and I wanted out. So I got out! How? I stopped stuttering severely with much less effort than I once used in trying in the wrong way to stop. And the wrong ways were to try to run from it, hide from it and forget it. I made the mistake of using every trick in the book to pretend to be a normal speaker, but none of the tricks worked for long. Failures only increased, and after years of agony I finally discovered that it was finally time to make an about-face. Why try to avoid and camouflage stuttering any longer? Who was I trying to fool? I knew that I stuttered, and so did my listeners. I finally took time out to ask myself why I should continue to fight the old, destructive feelings in the wrong way. I began to look at these feelings, and as I began to accept them and my stuttering, success in speaking began. It is interesting that the old ways of struggling were so difficult to give up. It felt as though I had an angry tiger by the tail and dared not let go.

I talked to the hearts of that excellent audience last evening and didn't pull my punches. Nobody should ever pull their punches when talking about the problem of stuttering. The problem is too vital to be treated in any other manner than with the truth. After the session was over I was gathering my notes together when I looked up and in front of me stood a young man in the throes of trying to say something. We shook hands and I listened and waited. A severe stutterer he was—so severe that apparently he dared not introduce himself. We sat down so that we might be as comfortable as possible, and in his unique pattern of speech, he asked some pertinent questions about himself and his stuttering.

The young man's first question had to do with whether there might be a physical cause for his stuttering. He explained that he was five years old when he was hit by a car and said that the scar was still on his neck. He wondered what other reason there could be to prevent him from saying his words fluently. To be struck by a car is a traumatic incident indeed, but I told this young man that his real scars were psychological ones and that the physical one on his neck was only skin deep. He was anxious to know what those psychological scars were and I was anxious to tell him that *he* knew better than *I*. "The answers lie in your looking closely at your stuttering pattern and at yourself."

This sincere young man asked a gut level question which all stutterers ask, "What do people think of me?" He said that he was weary of laughter and ridicule. I tried to explain that to a great extent he was putting the cart before the horse, the most important question that he should investigate is *what he thinks of himself*. I strongly suggested that he was by far his worst critic and that he had been living for years being his worst critic. But I also told him that he had lived most of his verbal life upon the judgments and misjudgments of others.

"It's your job," I emphasized, "to help other people understand. There's nothing like understanding that makes for the acceptance of differences. Help normal speakers to understand that what they are doing to stutterers is well-meaning, but wrong." I explained to him that we both knew that stuttering is indeed behavior which *is* different and that realistically we should not expect a person who has never had the problem to know what to do about it when he sees and hears it in another person.

I went further with this explanation because he was listening so intently. "When your listener looks away from you, it is because he thinks that you *want* him to look away. Ask him not to do it. It's as simple as this! When a listener laughs out of embarrassment, it might be tremendously helpful to realize that the embarrassment is the listener's, not yours. Don't borrow trouble, you've got enough of your own!"

We both agreed that the stutterer's listener should react to him just as though he is a normal person with an interesting kind of speech difference. That's how stutterers *want* to be treated, but they never request it. As a matter of fact, I had to tell him that *I* would feel more comfortable if he would look at me while we talked, and it was interesting that as he began to look at me he struggled less and less.

Now it was my turn to ask a question and I asked whether or not he thought that he had suffered long enough in feeling himself to be inferior. I indicated that his world of agony did not hinge solely upon his stumbling speech. His attitudes about himself, his listener and his speech were important. Hadn't he struggled long enough, and in vain, to pretend as best he could that he was not a stutterer? Be done with swinging at these straw men! They were *his* ghosts, not his listener's. I told him that his fear of stuttering is the greater part of the reason that he stutters. He seemed to understand.

It was my turn to ask still another question. "When was the last time you discussed your stuttering with anyone?" He said that he had never talked about it with anyone. "You know," I replied, "just as eye communication during speech is one of the most important ways to tell the other person that you have something to communicate, so is open discussion of your stuttering and your feelings about it." One of the biggest mistakes that stutterers and normal speakers make is to consider this problem to be a verboten, hush-hush subject.

I explained to this handsome young man (who had described himself as being repulsive) that no two stutterers stutter alike. Yet, every stutterer possesses two very strong and incapacitating feelings in common: *Fear* and *Anxiety*. Herein lies the heart of his problem. If the fear of stuttering can be reduced, then certainly stuttering itself can be reduced.

He wanted to know whether or not there would ever really be a cure for him. All stutterers search for the magic pill. I told him that a "cure" is rare, but not impossible. "But this doesn't mean that you have to live the rest of your verbal life in struggling. Why wrestle with those words so hard? You're even struggling between words," I pointed out to him. "You must be very tired!" He agreed that he was. Then I told him something else that gave him pause: "Don't make the mistake of trying to compete with others. Compete with yourself—from day to day, from speaking situation to speaking situation and from word to word. Competing with yourself means that you learn to understand *and cope with* the fears that surround your speech.

The young man told me that he knew of no place to go for help and some relief from his stuttering. I answered that it would be ideal if he could find some place and named a few university clinics where highly qualified speech clinicians with deep and intuitive understanding, work with stutterers. But I also emphasized to him that he could become his own speech clinician. He didn't get this idea right away, so I gave him some concrete suggestions.

"When a problem exists," I explained, "the first thing to do is to examine it carefully with the hope of discovering what was wrong." I told him that one of the most constructive things that he could do for himself was to observe himself several times a day in a mirror as he talked. Although it is a tough row to hoe at first, there is nothing as therapeutic as self confrontation. "Be as objective as possible," I found myself almost pleading with him. "Look and listen closely and discover just what it is that you are doing when you stutter. And after you make these discoveries, *refuse* to make them again. Easier said than done? Yup! But it's well worth every effort that you put into it. When you begin to *really* accept yourself as the stutterer you are, you're on your way to much easier speech and most certainly to greater peace of mind." I also suggested that he get himself a tape recorder and listen to himself with long ears. He'd soon discover that 90% of his stuttering consists of behavior that has made his stuttering more severe, not less severe.

The job is to think and work in a positive manner. The job involves coming to realize that those head jerks, eye blinks, tongue clicks, postponements on feared words, substituting non-feared words for feared ones, and the thousand and one ways in learning "how not to stutter" are not helping to get those words out. They are preventing the words from being said strongly, aggressively and fluently.

"Those blocks may look and sound like monsters to you now, but you can turn them into straw men. Attack them! You must *refuse* to allow your words and fears to control you. Remember that one failure leads to another and you're really trapped if you're caught in the web of misunderstanding the dynamics of your stuttering symptoms." He was listening intently.

"Know and remember that success begets success and self pity will get you nowhere!" Yes, he was still listening intently and was seeming to absorb the messages. Does working on yourself take guts? You bet it does! Does using your guts pay off? You bet it does!

My parting words to this young stutterer, in whom I hoped a wise investment had been made, were "Try it! You'll like it! . . . and let me hear from you."

And now, five cups of coffee later, I hope again that I have touched and helped another stutterer to help himself.

Desirable Objectives and Procedures For an Adult Stutterer

Wendell Johnson

I believe that as a "representative adult stutterer" you should look upon your "stuttering" as certain things which you have learned to do—not something that is "wrong with you" or that "happens to you." You should strive to substitute the normal speech behavior of which you are basically capable for the undesirable ways of reacting that you have learned.

Here is one basic method you can use. At a time when you feel that you "are stuttering" pay very close attention to what you are doing. A clinician can help you do this by asking you—or you can ask yourself—precisely what you are doing. You should answer this question in descriptive detail, and when you have done this you should ask yourself why you were doing what you were doing. Did you think you had to do these things? For what physical or other reasons? What good evidence do you have for the reasons you give? What did you hope to accomplish by doing those things? Did you think you had to do them in order to say what you wanted to say? Or "to keep from stuttering"? Would you talk better or worse if you did not do those things? If you did not do those things would you do more or less of something else, or nothing at all, that you would classify as "stuttering"? Would you be able to speak satisfactorily without doing those things? If not, why not? If so, why do you do them at all?

By means of this "practice in being clear about what you mean and how you know what you are talking about" you tend to find out that the doubts, fears, tensions, and related reactions that make up your "stuttering" are unnecessary and pointless, and that without them you speak all right. You tend to develop the conviction that what you call your "stuttering" is something that you do that you do not have to do and had better not do. It is made up of things you do trying not to do what you call "stuttering"—but they are themselves the "stuttering" you are trying not to do. In other words, "stuttering" is what you do trying not to "stutter" again. Why try to keep from doing something that you won't do at all if you don't try to keep from doing it?

On the basis of this conviction that your "stuttering" is made up of the things you do trying to keep from "stuttering" and that you can talk all right if you don't do these things, you become able to persuade yourself more and more effectively "to go ahead and talk." With this conviction, moreover, you will tend to regard the doubting, fearing, and tensing which you continue to do as error rather than abnormality. You will tend to think of these things as mistakes to be calmly taken in stride while you are making them, but not as mistakes that you can never stop making.

On this basis, you will be prepared to benefit from speaking as much as possible to more and more persons and in more and more situations. Meantime, you should continue to put yourself through the "what are you doing—why are you doing it—what else could you do if you didn't do it?" routine as often and for as long as you feel you benefit from it. In these ways you can develop more and more thoroughly the beliefs and feelings and reactions of normal speech.

You will achieve your objectives most readily with a qualified clinician who can help you obtain the information you need and discuss it with you; assist you in making the most of your practice activities and your observations of your own speech behavior and that of other persons; enable you to take part in individual and group learning experiences; listen sympathetically and understandingly when you want to talk about your problem and your feelings about it; and give you the advantage of any instruction and counseling that you may need.

Message to a Stutterer

Joseph G. Sheehan

If your experience as a stutterer is anything like mine, you've spent a good part of your life listening to suggestions, such as "relax, think what you have to say, have confidence, take a deep breath," or even to "talk with pebbles in your mouth." And by now, you've found that these things don't help; if anything, they make you worse.

There's a good reason why these legendary remedies fail, because they all mean suppressing your stuttering, covering up, doing something artificial. And the more you cover up and try to avoid stuttering, the more you will stutter.

Your stuttering is like an iceberg. The part above the surface, what people see and hear, is really the smaller part. By far the larger part is the part underneath—the shame, the fear, the guilt, all those other feelings that come to us when we try to speak a simple sentence and can't.

Like me, you've probably tried to keep as much of that iceberg under the surface as possible. You've tried to cover up, to keep up a pretense as a fluent speaker, despite long blocks and pauses too painful for either you or your listener to ignore. You get tired of this phony role. Even when your crutches work you don't feel very good about them. And when your tricks fail you feel even worse. Even so, you probably don't realize how much your coverup and avoidance keep you in the vicious circle of stuttering.

In psychological and speech laboratories we've uncovered evidence that stuttering is a conflict, a special kind of conflict between going forward and holding back—an "approach-avoidance" conflict. You want to express yourself but are torn by a competing urge to hold back, because of fear. For you as for other stutterers, this fear has many sources and levels. The most immediate and pressing fear is of stuttering itself and is probably secondary to whatever caused you to stutter in the first place.

Your fear of stuttering is based largely on your shame and hatred of it. The fear is also based on playing the phony role, pretending your stuttering doesn't exist. You can do something about this fear, if you have the courage. You can be open about your stuttering, above the surface. You can learn to go ahead and speak anyway, to go forward in the face of fear. In short, you can be yourself. Then you'll lose the insecurity that always comes from posing. You'll reduce that part of the iceberg beneath the surface. And this is the part that has to go first. Just being yourself, being open about your stuttering, will give you a lot of relief from tension.

Here are two principles which you can use to your advantage, once you understand them: they are (1) your stuttering doesn't hurt you; (2) your fluency doesn't do you any good. There's nothing to be ashamed of when you stutter and there's nothing to be proud of when you are fluent.

Most stutterers wince with each block, experiencing it as a failure, a defect. For this reason they struggle hard not to stutter and therefore stutter all the more. They get themselves into a vicious circle which can be diagrammed as follows:

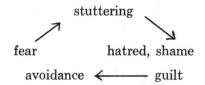

Stuttering is a lonesome kind of experience. Possibly you haven't seen too many stutterers and those you have seen you have avoided like the plague. Just as there may be people who know you or have seen you or even heard you who don't realize that there's anything wrong with your speech, so those who have a speech handicap similar to yours keep it concealed. For this reason few realize that almost one percent of the population stutter, that there are more than a million and a half stutterers in the United States today. That many famous people from history have had essentially the same problem, including Moses, Demosthenes, Charles Lamb, Charles Darwin, and Charles I of England. More recently, George VI of England, Somerset Maugham, Marilyn Monroe, and the T. V. personalities, Garry Moore and Jack Paar have been stutterers at some time in their lives. In your speech problem you may not be as unique or as much alone as you had thought!

Each adult stutterer has his individual style, made up usually of tricks or crutches which are conditioned to the fear and have become automatic. Yet they all suffer from basically the same disorder, whether they choose to call it stammering, a speech impediment, or something else. *How* you stutter is terribly important. You don't have a choice as to whether you stutter but you do have a choice as to how you stutter. Many stutterers have learned as I have learned, that it is possible to stutter easily and with little struggle and tension. The most important key in learning how to do this is openness: getting more of the iceberg above the surface, being yourself, not struggling and fighting against each block and looking your listener calmly in the eye, never giving up in a speech attempt once started, never avoiding words or ducking out of situations, taking the initiative in speaking even when doing a lot of stuttering. All these are fundamental in any successful recovery from stuttering.

You can stutter your way out of this problem. As long as you greet each stuttering block with shame and hatred and guilt, you will feel fear and avoidance toward speaking. This fear and avoidance and guilt will lead to still more stuttering, and so on. Most older therapies failed to break up the vicious triangle because they sought to prevent or eliminate the occurrence of stuttering which is the result of the fear. You can do better by reducing your shame and guilt and hatred of stuttering which are the immediate causes of the fear. Because stuttering can be maintained in this vicious triangle basis, there are many adults who could help themselves to speak with much less struggle if they would accept their stuttering, remain open about it, and do what they could to decrease their hatred of it.

Some individuals, given a start in the right direction, can make substantial headway by themselves. Others need more extensive and formal speech therapy or psychotherapy in clinics.

Because you stutter, it doesn't mean you are any more maladjusted than the next person. Systematic evaluation of objective research using modern methods of personality study show no typical personality pattern for stutterers, and no consistent differences between those who stutter and those who don't. Because you stutter, it doesn't mean you are biologically inferior or more neurotic than the next person. Maybe a little fortification with that knowledge will help you to accept yourself as a stutterer and feel more comfortable and be open about it.

If you are like most of the million and a half stutterers in this country, clinical treatment will not be available to you. Whatever you do you'll have to do pretty much on your own with what ideas and sources you can use. It isn't a question of whether self-treatment is desirable. Clinic treatment in most instances will enable you to make more systematic progress. This is particularly true if you are among those stutterers who, along with people who don't stutter, have personality and emotional problems. Every stutterer does try to treat his own case in a sense anyway. He has to have a modus operandi, a way of handling things, a way of going about the task of talking.

I have tried to set down some basic ideas which are sounder and more workable than the notions that most stutterers are given about their problem.

You might go about it this way. Next time you go into a store or answer the telephone, see how much you can go ahead in the face of fear. See if you can accept the stuttering blocks you will have more calmly so that your listener can do the same, and in all other situations see if you can begin to accept openly the role of someone who will for a time stutter and have fears and blocks in his speech. But show everyone that you don't intend to let your stuttering keep you from taking part in life. Express yourself in every way possible and practical. Don't let your stuttering get between you and the other person. See if you can get to the point where you have as little urge for avoidance and concealment in important situations as you would when you speak alone. And when you do stutter—and you will—be matter of fact about it. Don't waste your time and frustrate yourself by trying to speak with perfect fluency. If you've come into adult life as a stutterer, the chances are that you'll always be a stutterer, in a sense. But you don't have to be the kind of stutterer that you are—you can be a mild one without much handicap.

Age is not too important a factor, but emotional maturity is. One of our most successful recoveries on record is that of a 78-year-old retired bandmaster who resolved that before he died he would conquer his handicap. He did.

In summary, see how much of that iceberg you can bring up above the surface. When you get to the point where you're concealing nothing from your listener, you won't have much handicap left. You can stutter your way out of this problem, if you do it courageously and openly.

Helping Yourself Overcome Stuttering
Dominick A. Barbara

Speech is a fundamental aspect of the whole personality. Its function is not only to communicate verbally but also to express relationships. The stutterer never stutters when he sings or is in certain relaxed social situations. Instead, he has difficulty speaking whenever he comes in contact with certain forms of authority, or gets into situations where he feels his inner psychic balance and security are threatened.

If a stutterer wants to help himself stutter less, he must arrive at some understanding of *what* he is feeling and *what* he is meaning to convey to his listener, rather than *why* he is blocking. For example, when a stutterer says, "I'm stuck on a word, I can't go on talking," it isn't sufficient just to take this expression at face value. At this level it appears the person is having difficulty speaking, feels helplessly stuck, and can't seem to get past a particular feared or bugaboo word. However, upon closer examination, and at a deeper level, the stutterer can discover that the reason he blocks and continues to do so is that his fear of showing weakness or displaying verbal disruption is an embarrassing and humilating condition. Through stuttering he also reveals that his imagined omnipotence as a "flawless speaker at all times" is threatened; this ultimately leads him into potential failure and disapproval as a speaker.

Encouraging yourself to "speak up" or "to speak slowly" alleviates the problem only temporarily. You may attempt to control your stuttering by sheer will power, learn better devices for avoiding bugaboo words, or speak in a rapid manner in order to race through the possibility of stuttering. Only when you approximate inner balance with a healthy coordination of feelings and action can you rid yourself of your stutter and ultimately achieve relaxed and spontaneous speech. At first this may appear to be a difficult and impossible task, but with some degree of tolerance and self-discipline you can achieve at least the initial breakthrough to your inner problems, and to an ultimate resolution of stuttering.

The stutterer has a *Demosthenes Complex*. He makes demands upon his speech and his intellect which are excessive and impossible to achieve. This verbal perfectionism creates unnecessary inner chaos and turmoil. The person who tends toward stuttering feels he should *always* speak calmly, *never* appear ruffled, and *constantly* be in control of his listener. When he speaks he demands of himself the ultimate and the impossible. He feels he should be the master of his words and have a reservoir of everflowing facts and ideas. He should speak in a clear and concise manner, pause at the right time, never run ahead of his ideas, and be continually spontaneous and interesting when talking.

On the whole, people who stutter are highly intelligent and capable. Yet there appears to be a discrepancy between their realistic capacities and potentialities and what they unrealistically expect of themselves. Although there are many areas of productivity through which an individual can express his capacities and earn a comfortable living, I have found that many stutterers seem to be drawn toward jobs or professions where the use of verbal communication is paramount. It is not uncommon to find people who have difficulty speaking attempting to become salesmen, lawyers, psychologists, and radio announcers. There is no serious objection to this endeavor provided stuttering does not interfere too greatly. As a stutterer you can become successful in most jobs or occupations. However, to attempt to become a trial lawyer, where you would have to plead your case in court and be able to use your words in a forceful and astute manner, would be sheer folly for an active stutterer. The law profession offers many opportunities outside the courtroom for the use of abilities, knowledge and potentialities in the preparation of briefs, or other equally satisfying legal capacities, where speaking plays a minor role.

There are some "Do's and Don't's" that might help you work on your stuttering problem:

1. Since speaking is a healthy and volitional form of self-expression, the stutterer should encourage himself to "speak up" and "speak with others," not as a performance task, but as a means of arriving at social communion and communication. At first this will appear embarrassing and difficult, but the more you accept your shortcomings and the less you put emphasis on your impediment, the more relaxed you will become and the greater interest will you develop in self-expression.

2. Instead of depending on his natural resources for speaking, the stutterer generally resorts to various learned maneuvers,

evasions, substitutions, and magical rituals. He substitutes an "easy word" for a "feared word," adds extraneous words to help him over difficult spots, postpones the utterance of a sound by the use of "ah-ah," or even changes the entire context of what he is saying. These devices help the stutterer break through a hesitation or block, but they are basically artificial in nature and actually intensify the stuttering itself.

Get rid of these artificial devices! This may seem impossible or difficult at first, but depend upon your own natural resources and you will find that in the final analysis you will be greatly rewarded. Of course when you first attempt to relinquish these devices your stuttering will get worse; but if you have the patience, tolerance and courage to survive the initial blows, your spontaneous and normal speech will ultimately win over. Practice this a few minutes each day with your spouse, your parents or a trusted friend and you will be amazed at the results.

3. The stutterer is strongly dependent upon the reactions of his audience. What he fears depends to some degree on how he feels he will perform in the act of speech itself, and to a large extent, upon the response he expects from his listener. The stutterer is in constant need of the approval, praise, recognition and reassurance from other people. He feels that since he stutters he can make claims on other people for absolute understanding, sympathy, consideration and attention. Because of his heightened sensitivity to coercion, criticism, rebuff, or even the slightest denial, his listeners become constant threats to his particular problem. The more threatening his audience appears the greater the amount of rejection he will experience from others. The use of these claims upon others, based solely upon one's stuttering, is unrealistic and can only lead to frustration, repressed anger, and to perpetual entrapment.

To avoid this dilemma make your expectations more reasonable. Don't expect everyone to approve or accept everything you say. If more than half of what you say is accepted or agreed upon, you are running a good average. Don't expect everyone to blindly accept, love or admire you. Most people have problems of their own and may not have the capacity of becoming involved with you. Also remember that we listen to only 50 per cent of what we hear, and comprehend only 25 per cent. If you are operating within this range you are doing well. Finally, as you feel more confident and accept yourself and others more realistically, the less you will have the need to stutter.

4. One of the most important things for a stutterer to remember is get his feelings out into the open. There is plenty of room in discussions for agreement and disagreement, providing it can lead to productive communication.

Accept yourself! This is the key word to your verbal success. Accept both your assets and your limitations. When you feel important to yourself and equal to others, you no longer experience your speech as foreign, but as coming from somewhere inside of you.

When you feel yourself stutter, interrupt your speech, take control of yourself, and find a good balance within yourself. Forget that you have just had some difficulty and attempt some honest or jovial remark about it. Now you can start all over again with greater inner confidence and your chances of stuttering a second time are greatly reduced.

Do not become overwhelmed by a feeling of disaster. The embarrassment and humiliation you experience comes mainly from within yourself, and the feelings you think your listeners are experiencing are mostly fabrications of your own. Most listeners are interested in *what* you are saying, and should you stutter, they usually have compassion for your difficulty and overlook it in the face of continuing the relationship.

Finally, do not live through your words alone. You need not depend upon your words as your sole means of communication. The spoken word is merely a symbol of something else and does not carry with it an effect of dread or fear. Do not be afraid to use your words with courage and conviction. A careless word does not cause a calamity. The speaking situation should not be experienced as an arena of combat where one can emerge the victor or succumb to the mercy of others. In the final analysis, speaking should be considered as a means of verbal exchange with plenty of room for individual and mutual expression of thought, wishes, ideas and feelings.

Once you feel that you are in command of your own speech you will no longer feel hopelessly caught in its grip. Only then will you feel that you have a choice in whatever you are saying. Once you grow within yourself, the more courageous and confident you will feel as a human being. Finally, the less conflict you experience the more you will discard anything that is disturbing within yourself, including your stuttering. Energies which are utilized in the process of keeping your stutter alive are now freed to be used toward healthy growth and self-realization. You will become more relaxed, spontaneous, alive and productive. Speaking will now be used for the sole purpose of communicating and relating, and not as an area of testing.

Overcoming Fear and Tension
In Stuttering

JAMES L. ATEN

Most people talk without much difficulty most of the time. It's true that people hesitate and stumble over words at times, especially when under stress or fatigue, but they show little concern over such mistakes. What, then, makes your speech different and what can you do to help yourself? Invariably, the person who stutters overreacts to his mistakes. He fears they will occur, becomes tense and feels helpless. During the time that tension is so high, the flow of speech stops or will not start. As you continue to have these tense moments that become different from what normal speakers experience, fear increases to higher and higher levels. You come to dread and perhaps avoid speaking. Many stutterers learn that their greatest enemies are *fear* and *tension*. If the battle with stuttering is to be won, fear and tension must be gradually eliminated. Let's look at some battle plans that have helped quite a few stutterers conquer the majority of their fears, eliminate excessive tensions, and find that speech in most situations can once again come easily.

Conquering Fear. We have all probably heard that the way to eliminate fear is to "just face up to it." We have learned all too slowly that for some stutterers, fear may actually increase rather than decrease if they continue to face fear situations and fail. They may experience the same old tension, and fail to get the word out, while attempting to "just go ahead and face their fears." For most of you, fear grew because of repeated failure and the resulting embarrassment over that failure. Your *hope* is that fear can be unlearned by handling hard words and situations better. Performance builds *realistic confidence* that can become a substitute for fear. Here's one way: *Substitute Positive Planning for Fear and Anticipated Failure.*

Stuttering (the fear and tension build-up part) usually begins much earlier in time than you normally think. When the phone rings, you may get into a tense and helpless state while going to answer it. The trouble doesn't suddenly begin as you start to say "Hello." You have learned that tricks such as delaying or rushing often let you down and so your fear spirals upward. When told that you have a job interview in two days, you often begin worrying about how you'll do and expect failure. Having failed last time, you probably will again unless you plan a new approach to the task:

1. Picture yourself approaching the person who will be interviewing you. Take a breath, then *let* it all go. This feels good and for the first time you experience the condition your speech musculature should be in if words are to come out without tension.

2. Imagine extending your hand slowly to shake hands. Your body movements are slow and confident ones. This reduces the tendency to rush or force speech. Mentally you are calmer. The employer says "Hello, I'm John Wood. You must be . . ." Just thinking about answering this with your first and last name fills you with fear and you feel your breath tighten.

3. *LET GO* of that tight breath. Think about the easy movements you could make in answering "Hi, I'm Ed Jones." At first just picture the movements, then after that initial surge of fear subsides, try answering with a kind of easy, half-sigh-like *"Hi"*—Pause—easy again—"I'm *Ed*"—Pause again—let tension go—easy onset—"Jones."

As you rehearse this, several things begin to happen. First, you begin to see that there is less to fear if you don't jump and answer with your first name, which is usually very hard for you. Second, as one stutterer in our field has said, "Time must become your Friend." You will learn that "haste makes waste," even though a few times in the past it has worked.

Fear won't go away by just waiting or going slower; you have to do some positive planning and desensitizing yourself to the employer's presence and request. You must practice the introduction many times *and* not just alone but with someone. After you have experienced success alone, ask your wife or friend to be the employer and rehearse. First answer silently, then softly, then in a normal voice. Whether you stutter during the interview or not is of lesser importance. The chances are you will approach the situation easier than you have in a long time and that your actual stuttering will be less severe. New approaches to handling the feared situation bring gradual improvement by reducing fear. This comes through hard work, not magic, pills, tricks, or waiting until you "feel better." The same type of practice and rehearsal can be used in preparing to say "Hello" on the telephone. In fact, you may find the phone less fear-inducing and want to try it first, or, perhaps just greeting someone casually. As one stutterer said, "I try not to go out and put myself into a very difficult situation at first, where I know I'm going to fail." He had learned to approach some situations, though obviously not all of them, by thinking about responding the new easier, relaxed way and with practice found that he had lost much of his fear. Less fear means less tension in speech.

Conquering Tension. You must learn to substitute easy, slower, more relaxed movements for rushed, tight, forced movements. Typical tension sites are your chest and breath, your throat and vocal cords, jaw, lips and tongue. The practice suggested here can make for success in reducing the fear that follows from blocked movements, so think of these as stages of therapy that you can "put together" for greater effect.

Choose some words that begin with sounds that you think of as being hard—those on which you often stutter. Speech normally begins with a relaxed, unconscious flow of breath. Practice sighing and letting voice come easily. You don't make voice, it just happens if you will *let* it. The same is true of sounds you make with tongue and lips. Feel yourself gently close the lips for the "P" or move the tongue to form such sounds as "T" and "K", then go ahead and say the rest of the word. Notice how little effort speaking takes. Fear has resulted in too much forcing to get words out. You must learn what 'not forcing' is, and practice until easy movements become habitual. First, practice at a very soft, almost silent level, then gradually at a normal voice level. Practice the movement gently to make the difficult word begin easier, then work on other words that begin with that same movement. Assuming that you engage faithfully in daily practice, try a different sound each week. Fear of words lessens as you repeatedly prove to yourself you have a new, easy way of producing them that is becoming automatic. As you practice, be sure not to let the tongue, lips, vocal cords, or breath become tight or touch too hard. No word or speech movement requires conscious effort. Feel the relaxed easy movements into and out of words. *Stop* and begin the easy movements again for the next word series. Now, you are talking in phrases that are short and that you have confidence you can initiate, if you remember to use the easy beginning you have practiced. Remember, speech sounds better in short phrases with frequent pauses.

By conquering fear-arousal through learning to plan your approach, and then using the easy movements which keep tension from making you feel helpless, you are beginning to control stuttering rather than letting it rule you. Certain speaking situations become easier. At this point you must begin to integrate your success. That is, you are not just *having* good and bad days, you are creating some successes out of potential failure. That's what building confidence is all about—and stutterers say time after time, "I talk better when I'm more confident." When you have created a better performance, you can realistically feel more confidence. The model is then begun for turning 'bad cycles' into good ones. You are then able to turn your attention to fluency rather than frequent expectation of stuttering. One of our adult stutterers who successfully went through the above said, "Now I think more about my fluent successes, and does that ever help!"

You appreciate most in life those things you do for yourself. Getting over stuttering takes tremendous self-discipline and desire. We have found that just practicing easy movements without trying to reduce fear is not too successful, since high fear keeps you from remembering the new easier speech movements at the time when you most need to use them. Also, just trying to reduce fear without giving you something to do that is new— *and that works*—may simply allow fear to creep back into the situation very quickly. We have seen that the majority of the stutterers we work with, using the above procedures, achieve a significant degree of fluency in most situations.

Toward Freer Speech

FREDERICK P. MURRAY

Before embarking on the path of endeavoring to improve your speech, I suggest that you do some preliminary work along the lines of constructive and positive thinking. Motivation directed toward the goal of better speech is of the utmost importance if you are to move successfully along the road to better fluency. I would encourage you to tap whatever sources you have within you or might attain from religion, friends, or books, and utilize them toward this aim. Belief in yourself and cooperation with others are vital necessities as you undertake your task.

Do not expect the solution to years of confirmed stuttering to be rapid. Many stutterers have mistakenly believed that if only the "cause" could be found, a fast cure would result. Will the fire that is consuming a house extinguish itself merely because the match that started it has been discovered in an adjacent field? Stuttering in its advanced stages is self-perpetuating, much like a fire. It feeds on itself; fears of words and speaking situations act as cues to intensify it. Clearly, there will be a need for you to face up to, confront, and work upon your problem. This will call for active efforts on your part because strongly conditioned motor responses are changed by *action*, not by thought.

Many of you have heard about the wonders of hypnosis and may look to this technique to provide a quick answer. Rest assured that this has been tried throughout the years, but almost invariably with only temporary and fleeting success. It does not serve to build up the necessary resistance to the innumerable threats that now haunt you with regard to your oral communication. The ability to cope with these factors will come about only gradually as you change both your speaking behavior and personal attitudes, and as you adjust yourself to the new self-role that improved speech will thrust upon you. It is similar to an enormously fat man attempting to lose a hundred pounds. To do this safely he must do so at a rate that his heart and body can tolerate. If it occurs too rapidly, deep wrinkles will appear, and in extreme cases, he may collapse from the rapid change that his organism has undergone. The body needs a chance to integrate itself to each successive level of improvement in weight reduction. So it is with the stutterer who must adjust himself to better fluency. Therefore, I urge you to have tolerance with yourself as you proceed along the way. Do not demand the impossible at first! There is no law that states you must pick up the heavy end of the log everytime.

At this point it is appropriate to mention something about the likely dimensions of a recovery from a long standing bout with stuttering. It is highly improbable that you will ever be conscious of the month, or perhaps even the year, during which you master most of your difficulty. Specific steps of accomplishment along the way are hard to measure. You will, however, be able to cite a few key situations in which you surprised yourself by good performances and these will act as catalysts to your overall progress. Judging from my personal acquaintance with several dozen stutterers who have achieved a good recovery, I note there is not one who would claim to be completely fluent at all times. In other words, each one admits to occasional moments of disfluent speech or residuals of stuttering. However, persons who have not stuttered say that their speech fits approximately the same description. Some stutterers have arrived at a point where their overall speaking skill surpasses that possessed by the average speaker. So keep your head high!

Your ultimate goal, no matter how it may be reached, is to convince yourself that you are capable of speaking in oral communication situations. This is the opposite of saying to yourself that you cannot succeed in these situations because you cannot talk. The important thing, however, is that the conviction is thorough enough that it reflects itself automatically via your emotions and feelings. Remember, our speech is a mirror of how we feel at any given moment in time.

To help you in your goal the following guidelines are offered to provide information that should assist you.

Perhaps the first concrete step you should take is to acquaint yourself with your stuttering behavior. Odd as this may seem, few severe stutterers know what they are doing that interferes with the forward flow of speech. In order to carry this out effectively, you must first learn to keep in touch with yourself during your moments of stuttering. This is in direct contrast to attempting to run away from yourself and doing everything possible to try to avoid the occurrence of stuttering. Feedback of various types will assist you in this self-study endeavor. For example, you can look at yourself in a mirror and assess what you are doing while you make a phone call likely to elicit stuttering. Is it possible to record your speech in a communicatively stressful situation, then play the tape back for the purpose of careful analysis? Painful as this may seem, it is one good way to bring yourself to grips with your problem. If you can achieve a sufficient number of these behavior-exploring experiences you will discover that your stuttering is not a constant and fixed behavior; rather, it is something that varies greatly and is composed of some parts that are *not* handicapping. Regardless of the severity of the longer, highly abnormal blockages, each and every stutterer has some degree of easy moments of stuttering in his speech. These miniature stutterings represent goals in themselves. If you can learn to whittle the others down to similar proportion, more of your scoreable difficulty will have disappeared. This leads to the realization that there are countless ways in which to stutter. Even though you may have no choice as to whether or not you will stutter, you do have the choice of *how you stutter.*

It is also necessary to develop an awareness of the feelings you have in connection with your stuttering. Often your speech difficulty may seem to overwhelm you so much that you are unable to evaluate objectively the emotions that are intimately tied with it. Anxiety, guilt and shame are usually linked to severe speech blockages. Clearly, there will be a need to make some degree of separation between these compulsive forces. Success in accomplishing this should deprive the stuttering of some of its most powerful maintaining factors. Your fundamental task is twofold: alter your speech behavior, and bring about positive changes in your self-perceptions and feelings. A longstanding psychological principle states that one way to influence emotions and bring about a change in feeling is to deal directly with the outward behaviors that are associated with, and are the chief symptoms of, these inner states. If you can modify the severity of your more grotesque speech interruptions by substituting more relaxed forward-flowing speech movements, you will be putting this psychological principle into action. One excellent way to encourage this is by carefully planning certain speaking experiences. Your immediate goal should be to allow yourself to *stutter openly* and without tension and struggle. Do not try to speak as fluently 'as possible! By deliberately permitting yourself to prolong the initial sounds of many of the words you use, you will be taking the psychological offensive. You will be providing yourself with new outlets through which much of the built-up anticipatory fear can be dissipated, rather than steadily mounting up inside you. In addition, you will be giving your neurophysiological system an opportunity to work in better harmony rather than having one component counteract another. You will be confronting rather than avoiding your problem; the habitual avoidance of speech situations and feared words will get you *nowhere* in the long run. The sooner you are able to give up your holding-back behavior, the better! The following guidelines can serve to help you along the path of recovery from stuttering:

1. The handicap of stuttering consists mostly of learned behaviors. These can be unlearned.
2. Stuttering behaviors can be changed. Remember, you can choose how to stutter even if you cannot choose not to stutter.
3. A person can stutter in many ways.
4. Emotions can be altered by modifying symptoms associated with them.
5. Fear and avoidance lessen as confrontation is increased.
6. Long lasting improvement is unlikely to occur in a scientific laboratory setting. Learn to assemble your own portable laboratory and use it in the real world.
7. Recovery is probably going to be a long and gradual process. Have patience with, and respect for, yourself.

This summarizes and highlights what I have found to be an effective means of fostering improvement in speaking behavior, and maximizing the possibility of attaining a workable solution to your problem. Good Luck!

Change: Potential Qualities Become Actualities

Joseph G. Agnello

I stuttered very severely from the age of 3 years until the age of 28. What occurred during those 25 years with regard to my speech problem is another topic, but what brought on some of the miraculous changes in my speech and personal characteristics can be attributed to my therapist. However, the therapy under him did not bring on a great deal of immediate change in my speech performance. I still had repetitions and the forcing of syllables, but even so I was extremely satisfied when therapy was terminated. I felt I could *move forward in my speech.* I could speak whole sentences and phrases without getting severely hung-up on a syllable. This in itself was very satisfying to me and at that time was as good as being cured. Many of my peers and teachers did not understand how I could stutter so severely and yet talk on, almost oblivious of the tremendous amount of hesitations and blockings. What they failed to recognize was that I could now move forward in my speech. I was free to express all kinds of thoughts. I could even order a chocolate soda without being traumatized by the whole damn incident.

Prior to therapy I had many *preconceived and false ideas about why I stuttered.* Since so much advice is given so freely, and since none of the advice ever appears to do much good, one doesn't really feel there is much that can be done about stuttering. Some of the advice I received was good but I was not ready to make use of it, and consequently, I rejected it. Advice that one cannot act upon to bring about change is usually discarded forever, and in many respects this is too bad.

There are certain feelings and attitudes about stuttering that seem to perpetuate the problem. Most of them have little basis in fact. Some of the feelings and attitudes that plagued me during my early years were: I will always have this inability to talk; I stuttered because there was something wrong with my mind, because I was mentally slow, because nobody really liked me, because my father was a drunkard and was mean to me, because I masturbated, because I could not face up to my stutterings; I stuttered because I stuttered, because I was so nervous, and because I thought faster than I could talk, etc.

On the other hand, when I didn't stutter I thought it was

due to certain positive traits about me. Some of these were that I was a good athlete, was intelligent, had a good sense of humor, and was friendly. All of the "becauses" don't really make much sense. They don't offer any sensible explanations. For instance: Why those moments of severe stuttering? Why times of less stuttering? Why *any* fluency? WHY? To dwell on the "becauses" and "whys" only circumvents the reality of the problem.

After resolving some of these preconceived notions about my stuttering I felt free to try different things with my speech. I no longer felt bound to my old pattern of stuttering. I now felt a new ability to move forward and the feeling of personal freedom to explore and plan my own course of action. It was *self-confrontation to questioning that eventually brought on insights*. Questions such as How serious is my stuttering? Is my problem just stuttering or is it maybe not knowing how to relate to people? Do listeners really care if I stutter or is it the way I react to my stuttering that determines how they will react? What do people really think about my stuttering? Maybe I have a problem of listening? How do other people talk and listen? How do I listen to myself? Do I really hear my stuttering? Do I seriously attend to the meaning of words? Can I change?

Most people are kind, gentle and usually mean well. Usually people are interested in what you have to say. It is a big job to talk *with* people. The fact that you get stuck on words is another issue. Even if you didn't get stuck on words you would still have an awesome responsibility in learning how to explain things clearly. *Speech is a public affair.* You must work on speaking forthrightly and clearly, and on establishing verbal relationships with other people. Think clearly of how you are going to say what you want to say and plan how you will organize your discourse. Think critically about your listener. What is his background? Does he understand what I mean? Am I going too fast for him? Is he afraid of me, or am I afraid of him? Why does he appear not to be listening to me? Is it my manner of talking? What can I do to make the listener more relaxed?

As a researcher I have spent many hours observing other stutterers and have made acoustical and physiological analyses of "how stutterers stutter." This was helpful to me because it forced me to examine my own stuttering very critically. I was fascinated by the peculiar ways I approached certain words and how I moved from one syllable to the next. Observations of my own stuttering and hard experimental work have led to what I think is the most universal feature concerning the basic problem stutterers exhibit with regard to the motor performance of speech production.

Timing is most crucial for on-going forward-moving speech. Voicing has to be precisely terminated and initiated at some point during the production of speech. Voicing must interact in a precise manner with articulatory movements and this is the likely site of difficulty. The glottal signal excites the oral cavity and an articulatory gesture must act to facilitate, check or terminate the glottal pressure. Any action that emphasizes or enhances *smooth transitions* from sound to sound, syllable to syallable, or word to word will be beneficial for on-going speech. Beyond the matter of word transition there is another form of stuttering that may be prevalent but not so obvious. This is stuttering on organization of thoughts. One thought concept must have organization with a transitional phase into the next thought. These thought units generally are encompassed within phrases. Any effort that disrupts, discourages, or fails to assist smooth transition will generally be identified as stutterings or eventually evoke a poor pattern of on-going "free speech."

I found the following practices to be helpful in my efforts to improve my speech:

1. Practice speaking in rhythm to a definite beat.
2. Practice speaking in the style of a famous speaker. Carl Sandburg spoke slowly, prolonged vowels and had long pauses. He was my model.
3. Fake stuttering. Make an effort to relate to some of the questions previously mentioned (Do I really hear my stuttering? and, How serious is my stuttering? etc.) When you fake stuttering with some objectives and questions in mind, you must assume responsibility both for yourself and for your listener. If the "fake stuttering" becomes "real" or you fail to be objectively critical about your stuttering, then you are most likely not being truthful to yourself and the listener.
4. Talk slowly and deliberately. Stutter slowly and deliberately.
5. Listen to recordings of your speech.

6. Use "loose pullouts" after getting stuck on a syllable. Come out of stuttering in an easy manner without the sudden jerks and plosive efforts.

7. Speak honestly to others about stuttering.

In summary, I feel the following developments were most instrumental in my acquiring what I consider to be "cured stuttering."

1. Giving up efforts to explain my stuttering and its causes. Too many "becauses" and false ideas about "why" I stuttered had only confused me and made things worse.

2. Organizing what I wish to say and organizing my manner of saying it so I can *move forward* in my speech, even if there is some stuttering.

3. Answering some very pertinent questions about my speech and myself through some serious self-confrontations.

4. Assuming the responsibility for talking and remembering that there is another person in the conversation, too. Learning to restrain myself and reserving judgments about myself and others. Learning to pause, to sit quietly, and listen attentively.

5. Working on actual speech exercises, tasks and assignments that were aimed at developing smooth articulatory co-ordination (motor planning) and transition from sound to sound, syllable to syllable, word to word, phrase to phrase, and thought to thought. Doing these tasks both alone and in real speaking situations.

Suggestions For Self-Therapy For Stutterers

Margaret M. Neely

Dear Fellow-Stutterer: If you are an adult who has stuttered most of your life, you have probably tried many ways to cope with the problem. So have I. As a stutterer and a therapist, my observation is that each person finds his own way. There are a multitude of approaches to the correction of stuttering. The procedure I suggest is not necessarily the "best" approach; it is simply an approach that has been effective for me and for most of the individuals with whom I have worked. It is a direct attack on the speech and it involves effort. Many people resist the work aspect and want easier ways to overcome the problem. The feelings of anxiety that accompany stuttering have become so overwhelming that the stutterer reacts by wanting a simple way with immediate results. Drug therapy to relieve anxiety and mechanical devices to block your own hearing or to supply you with rhythmic patterns are easy methods which seem immediately beneficial. I believe that nothing succeeds on a long term basis like hard work on the speech itself, an idea that may be due to the very personal viewpoint of anyone who is both a therapist and a stutterer. My own experience has been that nothing "cures" an adult stutterer but one can effectively manage stuttering so that it ceases to be a significant problem throughout one's life.

Why does this approach require work? Because speech, like walking and other body functions, is acquired early in life and becomes habitual long before school age. Those of us who stutter have learned both fluent and stuttered forms of speech which have become automatic. You, as a stutterer, must study your speech patterns in order to become aware of the differences between stuttered and fluent speech. Stuttered forms of speech can be changed in various ways, just as handwriting can be modified. It is this changing of an established habit that requires work.

Several psychological problems confront the stutterer as he tries to alter his speech. These problems include a lack of confidence in his ability to do anything with his stuttered speech because of previous failures, an inability to cope with feelings of resentment and loneliness about having this problem (why me?), and worry and concern about the effect of his stuttering on other people and their possible resulting opinions of him. In addition, the stutterer struggles with the idea that because he can say his words fluently some of the time, he should be able to say them fluently all of the time. He may believe some psychological problem needs to be removed and this belief results either in periodic over-worry about his speech or complete disregard for it. These feelings which have become automatic, as has the stuttering, usually are the painful part of stuttering. This is why you may feel the need to first work on eliminating the feelings you experience when you stutter. However, it is easier to work on the speech first, and the feeling next, because much of the accompanying emotion disappears when you have gained control of your speech.

How do you start?

Your goal should be to find a way of speaking that is comfortable for you. You will need to eliminate the abnormality of your stuttering and try to find an easier way to talk which is under your control.

Study your speech. Learn to change the habitual form of stuttering to a more controlled pronunciation of the word. Change your speech to include fluent speech, pauses and the controlled saying of words, as well as occasional stuttering.

To study your speech, analyze how you say words both fluently and in a stuttered form. You may think of a word as being a unit or "lump" of sound; actually a word is composed of separate sounds, much as a written word consists of separate letters. To say a word you must move from sound position to sound position with your speech articulators shaping the air that carries the voice. Learn to be aware of the feeling of muscle action as you move through a word. When a word is said fluently these muscular movements are coordinated, loose and easy.

When you stutter, you will notice that there is a great deal of tension in the speech muscles used to say the beginning sound. Much of the abnormality of stuttering is your automatic reaction to the feeling of the sudden muscle tension that you experience as a "blocked" feeling. You try to fight the blocking by pushing harder, rather than by releasing the tension and moving to the rest of the word. As you say an isolated word beginning with a B or P, for example, concentrate on the feeling of movement as you bring your lips together and as they move to the next sounds. In the habitual stuttering pattern the muscles will either tighten and then release to bounce back to the same position, or will jerk forward to the rest of the word. This is in contrast to a fluent saying of the first sound which will have loose contact of the lips and a smooth shift to the next sound position.

Study your conversational speech. You may stutter more in connected speech than when you say single words. Such factors as the speed of speaking and word position in a sentence can influence how a word is said, and can precipitate stuttering. Stutterers have a good deal of fluent speech as well as stuttered speech. Learn to be aware of the feeling of fluency and the sensation of fast, easy movement of the muscles involved in speech. These movements are interrupted only to take a breath, or to pause for meaning. When a pause for stuttering occurs, you may notice that the rate of speech increases after the block as if to "make up" for lost time. Sometimes this increased speed produces a rapid, jerky speech pattern that is difficult to understand. Stutterers usually hurry in their speech more than normal speakers do. You may want to consider changing the rate of both your fluent and your stuttered speech.

How do you practice changing the habitual form of stuttering to a controlled pronunciation of words?

Begin with single words. Watch in a mirror as you place your mouth in position to say the first sound of the word. Move slowly and gently from sound to sound through the word. Practice this silently, whispering, and then aloud as you learn to feel the sensation of relaxed movements of the lips, tongue, and throat. Through awareness of muscle movement you can control your speech production even when talking to other people and are unable to use a mirror.

Read aloud to yourself. Say each word in the sentence as if it were an isolated word. Be highly conscious of the feeling of movement through the word.

Practice saying words directly using a talking-and-writing technique. Write the first letter of the word as you begin to say the word and prolong the first sound until you have completed the written letter. This slow first movement of the word will train you to combat the excessive muscle tension which automatically occurs at the beginning of stuttered words.

Try to learn a new speech pattern which can be used in

every day speaking. You may have noticed that one of the important factors which influences the amount of stuttering in your everyday speech is your feeling of inner stability. This feeling is what you experience as self-confidence, calmness and self-control. Many influences from the environment, or from your physical state, can affect your equilibrium. Most of these environmental influences are beyond your control. However, you can change to a speech pattern that is under your voluntary control, rather than responding to the pressures with habitual tense and stuttered speech. This pattern should consist of your fluent speech, which you refuse to hurry, and your careful, relaxed, controlled speech. By using your awareness of muscle movement to guide your lips, tongue, and throat from sound to sound throughout the word, much as in writing, you can reduce much of the abnormality and tension that occurs in a stuttered word. Use of this controlled pronunciation on some of the fluent words as well as the stuttered words can keep a smooth speech pattern. This takes work, but can become habitual in many situations. Your over-all goal is to find a way of speaking that is comfortable for you. This should include the following ideas:

1. Acceptance of the idea that you are a "controlled" stutterer rather than a fluent speaker.
2. Awareness of the "feel" of shaping words fluently.
3. Mastery of the panic of stuttering will occur when you accept, as normal for you, the pauses and moments of tension that occur in your speech. By reducing the struggle of stuttering you relieve yourself of embarrassment, but you cannot hurry when stuttering.
4. Self-discipline in daily practice.
5. Humor as you look at your mistakes in speaking. Many things about stuttering can be funny.

Stuttering is a life-long problem which improves with age. As a stutterer you can gain great satisfaction in watching yourself acquire better and better control of speech as you work on it.

Self-Improvement After Unsuccessful Treatments

HENRY FREUND

Like most adult stutterers in this country you have probably been subjected to some form of therapy at one time or another. This therapy was either totally ineffective or resulted in only temporary improvement. Maybe it even resulted in a "cure," only to be followed by a relapse. Such an experience may have provoked in you an attitude of pessimism as far as the possibility of a more effective treatment is concerned. Or, it may have strengthened your desire for the "miracle," the perfect cure which would eradicate every trace of stuttering. Both these attitudes are unjustified.

For those who are pessimistic about the possibility of help it may be encouraging to learn that some stutterers have been able to help themselves either in spite of, or possibly because of, repeated and unsuccessful treatments. Some of the contributors to this book will give you specific and practical advice about what to do in times of trouble. I want to give you a short description of my own attempts at self-improvement, after many unsuccessful treatments, and the principles on which they were based. This is my own strictly personal way of helping myself and should not be considered as a blueprint to be followed rigidly. Each individual must go his own way.

For those who are overly optimistic a few words of caution are needed. I am intentionally talking only about *improvements* and not about *cures*. I am of the opinion that for the adult stutterer the best we can expect is long-term, even lifelong improvement, which renders him a less unhappy and less socially withdrawn person. This is not a perfect cure. Traces of the disorder usually remain and relapses occur. This applies equally to those who were treated by others and to those who treated themselves. It seems to me that those "former stutterers" who really don't have any trace of stuttering left did not recover as a result of planning and conscious efforts but actually outgrew their disorder without knowing how and why. Their cure is, as we say, a spontaneous recovery and not the result of therapy.

I was definitely a severe stutterer and was treated unsuccessfully by leading European authorities during my elementary school and high school years, as a student in medical school and even after graduation. Without the knowledge I acquired as a result of all these futile attempts at therapy, however, I probably never would have succeeded in helping myself overcome the worst of my stuttering. As an eight year old child I experienced a short-lived and almost miraculous improvement by using a smooth, melodic manner of speech with prolonged syllables; sentences were uttered as units. It was a manner of speech akin to singing. I noticed that I could apply this method in front of strangers with perfect ease and confidence when accompanied by my therapist. But he accompanied me only rarely, and never made any systematic attempt to enlarge the range of situations I could master. I returned home as "cured," only to relapse quickly. The next two authorities conducted therapy strictly within the walls of their office. The first one, after many tricks and much logical persuasion, finally stumbled upon rhythmic speech; again I felt an almost miraculous ease, but no attempt was made to help me apply this in front of others. The last therapist totally rejected my request to accompany me into real life situations. He wanted me to have the courage to do it alone. My numerous attempts to approach people alone and to con-quer my fear of stuttering all ended in failure and my stuttering grew worse. From bitter experience I learned how futile it is to make demands upon the stutterer without giving him a helping hand. What I needed was not an authority but a friend and collaborator genuinely interested in me and ready to help me. I was fortunate to have a brother who could be this friend.

At age 35 I gave up my practice as general practitioner of medicine and moved from Yugoslavia to Berlin for postgraduate training and specialization. My shyness to approach people had reached a point where something had to be done about it and I was now given an opportunity to make a new start and my chances for a successful attempt at treating myself were favor-able. Not only had I accumulated an extensive knowledge on stuttering, but through my many unsuccessful treatments in the past I had developed definite ideas of what was necessary to do to bridge the gap between theory and practice. I tried to follow these main principles.

1. I determined to make full use of the opportunity to devote myself completely to the task of self-improvement. The

chances of success would be better if I were able to live completely for this one task. I had to make full use of a new environment where nobody knew me as "stutterer" and where nothing reminded me of my past defeats and humiliating experiences.

2. I knew by now that I possessed a normal ability to speak. Speaking is an automatic act and most of the time I did speak normally. I knew that stuttering occurred situationally, that it resulted from fear and the expectation of failure and that this lead to an inhibition or stoppage of the voice. I talked under the illusion that speech sounds are difficult and that an enormous amount of force was necessary to overcome my self-created obstacles. Talking was a highly emotional experience which gave me a feeling of helplessness, failure and defeat. But I also knew that the method I used as a child which stressed all the positive aspects of speech (the stream of breath and voice, the unity of the sentence as a whole, the singing-like, melodic aspects of speech) was in the past prone to draw my attention away from the dreaded speech sounds, tended to calm and relax me, and rendered my speech more pleasurable. As a first step I would now start again to use this method with those persons closest to me and regain my old confidence in it. I could use this as a steppingstone to contacts with others.

3. I would discuss with my brother my daily predicaments, fears, doubts, successes, defeats and other personal problems. After establishing a good and trusting relationship I explained my strategy. He should accompany me wherever and whenever I needed his help; he should remain silent when I was sure of myself but should take over when I stumbled; or he could start to talk and then I could gradually take over. In this manner I could slowly expand the variety of people and situations where I could talk methodically, calmly and confidently.

4. After establishing a greater degree of security and confidence I would be able to reduce and finally discard the need for my brother to accompany me. I would be on my own and would expand the range of situations I wanted to master. I would do this gradually and would not ask for too much too soon. In times of trouble, I should not be too proud to discuss my problems with others.

5. Having widened somewhat the range of situations and

people that I could handle without fear I had to secure my newly won abilities by preparing myself for the inevitable reversals. Relapses would be unavoidable and had to be expected for there would be no foolproof method to eliminate them. In the past relapses were prone to shatter my belief not only in a certain method, but also in ever being able to overcome my stuttering. This would not happen again if I were prepared to meet them in the right spirit. Situations and circumstances would arise when the magical power of any method would be overpowered by old fears and self-doubts, and when some outposts of the liberated area might get again lost. The right spirit to meet relapses and reversals is a philosophy of self-tolerance, of the acceptance of your own weaknesses and limitations, and of a greater objectivity toward self and others. This results in a lessened sensitivity. Here, too, an open discussion with an understanding person sometimes helps to clarify issues which subjectively you are unable to see clearly.

I followed these and other similar guidelines. The break-through occurred when, after a period of preparation and ac-companied by my brother, I for the first time dared to approach a stranger for the purpose of experimenting on him. In spite of a panic-like fear and desire to run away, I heard myself asking him a question in a surprisingly calm and methodic fashion. This first breakthrough shattered the walls of fear and avoid-ance. It was a positive emotional experience of strong impact; it created a new confidence and opened up new vistas. The world became a friendlier place to live in and I felt closer to other human beings. Many similar positive experiences followed. My liberated verbal territory became too big to ever again fall prey to the demons of fear and doubt. For the next six years I spoke practically without conscious fear of stuttering and was able to engage in activities like counseling, lecturing and teaching as head of several speech clinics. These tasks I could not have possibly performed before. Then minor relapses, especially dur-ing exceptionally difficult life-situations, started to occur. While traces of the disorder have remained, and while with advancing age I have again become slightly more socially handicapped, the disorder never again assumed the severity it had prior to age 35. But even now, 40 years later, I still not only continue to study myself but also to treat myself. I still work to normalize my relationship to others and on my life-philosophy. For me, this is a lifelong task.

This is my story of self-improvement after unsuccessful treatment. Maybe there are some ideas which will prove helpful to you. I hope so!

Some Helpful Attitudes Underlying Success in Therapy

Harold L. Luper

It's been more than twenty-five years since I first entered the speech therapy program which proved effective in significantly reducing my speech problem. Much has happened in speech pathology since that time. Although there have been few completely new techniques, the manner of programming these techniques and the manner in which they are applied to persons have continually been improving. Speech pathologists are constantly seeking better ways to help the stutterer and what's considered best today will probably be replaced in the future with something better. For this reason, I shall not dwell as much on the specific techniques and activities that helped me as upon the general attitudes and principles which seem to underlie successful stuttering therapy.

The Power of Constructive Assertiveness. A few years ago, Norman Vincent Peale popularized a set of attitudes in his book, *The Power of Positive Thinking*. One of the principles that I found of most value in changing my stuttering problem might be called *constructive assertiveness*. Like many of you, one of the most common and most debilitating characteristics of my problem was my habit of avoiding. I continually searched for ways to get around saying words on which I expected to stutter. There was almost no limit to what I would do to avoid situations in which I feared my stuttering would embarrass me. Going to a party would be an extremely tiring event because the entire evening would be spent trying to stay alert for words on which I might stutter and finding ways to avoid saying them.

Fortunately, even before I began active therapy, I found out that avoidance only makes the fear worse. While serving in the army, I had written a speech pathologist asking for help. He informed me he would be glad to see me after I was out of the service and gave me a few suggestions as to what I could do in the meantime. His most important suggestion was to begin to lick the problem of avoidance. He suggested I go ahead and say those words on which I expected to stutter and to go ahead and enter those situations which I normally avoided. I began to try it. It was hard, but soon I found that the temporary discomfort of struggling through a difficult word was far better than the constant vigilance and search for the easy way out. Through the years, I have found that this is still one of the best ways to reduce my anxiety and to improve my speech when I again begin to have trouble.

Being assertive means being aggressive. You don't need a therapist to harness this power. Search for those words or situations that are beginning to bug you rather than hiding them until they build up to giant fears. If you stutter on a particular word, you can deliberately use the word again in other conversations until the fear is gone. If a certain situation makes you tense so talking is difficult you can go back into similar situations until you feel more at ease. Where you used to avoid, search for positive constructive ways to reduce your fear and struggle. At times, it means bearing some temporary embarrassment while you stick it out on a hard word, but overall you'll find that your fear, tension, and struggle are less when you practice constructive assertiveness.

Exploring the Dreaded Unknown. Early in my therapy program, I made a startling discovery. Although I had stuttered for years, I really did not know much about what I did with my speech apparatus as I stuttered. Like many other persons who stutter, I had been so embarrassed when I was stuttering, that my total attention was drawn to trying to "get out of" my seemingly helpless struggle against an unexplainable "block." In therapy, my clinicians helped me learn to study my speech behaviors and to analyze what I was doing at those moments when I was struggling. Many of the things I was doing interfered with fluency more than they helped. Although in the past, I'd repressed awareness of my stuttering behaviors, I now found that much was to be learned from encountering and analyzing them. You, too, can explore the unknown. When you do, you may find that you push your lips together too hard or jam your tongue against the roof of your mouth. You may notice that as you start to say a word, you build up too much tension. Once you begin to see what you are doing that makes talking difficult, you find that much of this behavior is controllable. Concentrate on changing what you do when you stutter by doing differently some of the things that seem to interfere with your fluency. Stuttering will then lose some of its magical powers and become only those things which you do. Eventually you should make a very important discovery; that is, that you are not completely helpless at the moment you are stuttering.

Defining Realistic Obtainable Goals. Another helpful attribute that ties directly into the changes we've just been discussing is to set for yourself realistic and definable goals. Many of you will have, as I did, a rather perfectionistic attitude toward speaking. I wanted complete fluency with absolutely no stuttering. Anything less was a failure.

When you realize that all speakers have some hesitancy and disfluency in their speech, and when you realize that it is unrealistic to expect to change completely and immediately a problem you've lived with for years, you will be able to get satisfaction from small gains and to have greater tolerance for those difficulties you still encounter. Rather than hoping for complete fluency in each situation, work towards more realistic goals of improvement in certain specific behaviors, such as reduction of excessive lip tensing.

Reducing the Importance of Stuttering. One of the hardest things for me to learn was that the problem of stuttering is not the worst thing that can happen. For years I had felt stuttering was the biggest problem in life and this affected my entire self-perception. I was definitely handicapped because I was a member of the small minority that stuttered. Getting older has many disadvantages but it had the advantage of helping me put things in perspective. As I encountered other persons with other problems, I eventually realized that there are many difficulties worse than stuttering. One can still do most of what he wishes even if he does stutter.

Putting stuttering in a more realistic perspective may reduce some of your tension and make it easier for you to work on it. You should feel less embarrassed when it does occur, and you can stop thinking of yourself as a handicapped individual and thus improve your overall self-confidence.

Maintaining Improvements. Many of you who stutter have had the experience of getting better during therapy only to find yourself having trouble again when therapy is discontinued. This event, sometimes called a relapse, frequently leads to demoralization and the failure complex—a feeling that there's little use in trying to change your stuttering since it will probably return.

Frequently the person who has had this experience over-reacts to the return of struggle behaviors. He may well forget that even the amount of trouble he is having now is not nearly as frequent nor as severe as it was formerly. The fear of stuttering suddenly reappears and avoidance and struggle behaviors soon follow. Rather than accept this defeatist attitude, it's far better to go back to the basic principles; that is, determine what specific things you're doing and start again to do those things which you've found make talking easier.

Too many persons who stutter stop too soon after gaining some fluency and losing some of the fear. They fail to realize that stuttering behaviors have been learned on a complex reinforcement schedule over a long period of time. They fail to do those things which will maintain the new speaking behaviors. In all kinds of learning we normally go through three stages: (1) establishment of the new habit, (2) transfer of the habit to different situations, and (3) maintenance of the new behavior. If, after making some positive changes in your speech behavior, you revert to those attitudes and practices that originally were a part of the problem, you may find that the problem reappears.

To maintain the progress you've made in therapy it's wise to enlarge your speaking horizons. Now's the time to take that course in public speaking you've always dreaded or to begin to accept more invitations to social events where you know you'll have to meet a lot of people. Just as it's difficult to imagine maintaining recently learned swimming skills when you don't continue to go swimming, it seems pretty hard to imagine maintaining newly acquired attitudes and behaviors in speaking if you don't continue to enter a lot of speaking situations.

I hope some of my experiences will be helpful to you. Before ending, however, I must express a sincere debt of gratitude to the two persons who served as my clinicians some twenty-five years ago. They know who they are. I probably could have made many of the changes I've made without them, but I'm convinced they helped change my life for the better.

What You Can Do About Your Stuttering

J. DAVID WILLIAMS

You can do quite a bit if you really want to. You should begin by facing and describing those feelings and behaviors that make up your overall stuttering problem. Unless you know your problem in detail you won't know what you're working on or how much progress you've made. As honestly as you can, try to observe yourself and write down your observations. Then you can look at your own words. You may want to revise them later. Here are some questions you might try to answer.

Exactly what are your *feelings* about yourself as a stutterer and how do they affect your day-to-day relationships with other people? How do you feel when you know you're going to have to speak in various situations, how do you feel when speaking (during stuttering as well as not stuttering), and how do you feel afterward? What problems can you *really* blame on your stuttering? What are your stuttering *behaviors*? Use a mirror and a tape recorder to analyze yourself (this can be tough!). How much do you tense up and struggle when you start feeling "blocked" on a word? Do you compress your lips or hold them wide open, jam your tongue in certain positions, hold your breath, shut your eyes, or what? In which speaking situations do you do these things with the most tension? When *don't* you do them? During how much of your speaking time, or on about what percentage of your words, do you *not* stutter? To that degree you are a normal speaker. Keep that in mind! Your job is to change your feelings and behaviors so that you will speak *more* of the time the way you now speak some of the time. Quite possibly you're more of a nonstutterer than you are a stutterer.

You do not like your stuttering and its real or imagined social consequences, so it is natural to try to avoid it. At times you may totally avoid stuttering by choosing to be absent, by withdrawing from a speaking situation, or while speaking you may substitute a non-feared word (one on which you do not expect to stutter) for a feared one. This allows you to escape for the moment, but increases your worry about future situations.

What happens at the actual moment of stuttering and how do you react to the sudden feeling of blockage or paralysis? You may have a fairly simple, straightforward pattern of stuttering, or you may instantly swing into a tense performance of struggle behaviors. Can you determine what they are from your self-observations? You are struggling to be fluent and to avoid stuttering. Ironically, these struggle behaviors are what other people see and hear as your stuttering! You have sabotaged and double-crossed yourself. Your pattern of stuttering behavior consists chiefly of the things you are doing to avoid stuttering. That's a pretty basic idea. Mull it over a bit.

Instead of tense, out-of-control struggles, you need speech behaviors that don't try for impossibly perfect fluency but which do lead to good feelings of control, confidence, self-respect and decreased anxiety and frustration. These interfere less with communication and are more acceptable to you and your listener. So here they are! No tricks, gimmicks, secret recipes or instant cures; just voluntary modifications of your speech behaviors that will help you do what needs to be done.

Slow Stuttering. Do *not* change your usual rate of speaking unless you really speak too fast to be understood (very few people do). Leave your non-stuttered speech alone. But when you start to tense up and stutter, *at that instant* shift into slow motion. Don't give up your speech effort, but try to do everything easily, gently and slowly. Relax and let go; keep your lips, tongue and jaw moving without jamming. Don't panic. Take all the time you need; keep things moving slowly. Keep your confidence and don't buckle. Keep going forward slowly but positively. Totally resist any feeling of hurry or pressure. Let 'em wait. At some critical point in time (a second or less, two seconds, ten seconds or more) you will suddenly know you're over the hump. You'll feel your tension drain away as your confidence surges back. Simply finish that word and keep talking along at normal speed until you start to tense up for another bout of stuttering. Then you instantly shift into slow motion again.

Many stutterers who originally had very tense, complex patterns of stuttering have worked themselves down to this easy, simple, slow stuttering with little tension or interruption in their speech.

Sometimes a moment of stuttering seems to catch you by surprise, and you find yourself holding your mouth wide open or jamming your lips together as you feel the sudden surge of tension that leaves you frozen with panic and frustration. *Stop struggling* at that instant. Don't try to change your lip or tongue position. Hold everything as is until you feel your tension start to fade. Either keep the sound going, or gently re-initiate the sound you wanted to make; make absolutely no effort to finish the word until you can do so with complete ease. Then finish the word naturally and keep on talking. In this way you are deliberately taking control of the situation and are manipulating the behavior that has always seemed to be out of control.

Deliberate Repetition of Initial Sound or Syllable. At the first feeling of tension and struggle say only the first sound or syllable of the word easily and lightly, repeat it a few times until you feel relaxed and confident, then finish the word. "Please pass the sa-sa-sa-salt." If you start to tense up while repeating the sound or syllable, try to relax and let go again; keep the repetition going until all tension drains away, then perhaps toss in one or two more relaxed repetitions just to show yourself that you're in control before you finish the word. Remember, this is not real stuttering which is tense, struggling, out-of-control behavior. This is calm, relaxed, controlled, deliberate disfluency, and is a means of dissipating your tense, panicky feelings of impending stuttering.

Deliberate Repetition of Entire Word. Occasionally when you stutter on a word, really mess it up, and don't seem to be able to do anything about it at the moment, go ahead and stutter your way through it. After you complete the word, *stop!* Resist the tremendous urge to keep talking and pretending that your stuttering never happened. You need to confront the fact that it *did* happen. Go back and say the word over again, and again, and again, and more times if necessary until you say it easily and naturally with no tension. *Then* keep on talking. This leaves you with a feeling of success for having done something positive to conquer your fear and avoidance of stuttering.

In learning and practicing these behavior modifications, as in everything you do to work on your stuttering problem, you should proceed from easier tasks and situations to harder ones. Begin by practicing each of these techniques a few minutes daily in the easiest, least-threatening situation for you—either when alone or with someone else, and if possible with a mirror and tape recorder for visual and auditory "feedback." Approach doing them with calm confidence and relaxation. These behaviors may feel strange at first, but keep in mind *why* you are doing them, and with continued practice you will do them more easily, naturally and successfully. Always resist the urge to hurry or to pop the word out as quickly as possible. Panic, tension, and an overwhelming urgency are the hallmarks of stuttering; they are what you must overcome. Sooner or later you will begin to decide which of the behaviors best serve to give you a feeling of ease and confidence in speech, and reduce your tensions and your urge to fight your stuttering.

I would recommend the almost constant use of a tape recorder. There's nothing like being able to hear your own speech in order to judge what you do and don't like about it, and to decide what changes to make as you practice. Try to record your speech in different speaking situations. A small battery-powered recorder may be used in "real life" situations.

On separate index cards, list various speaking situations in which you fear stuttering. As you gain confidence in your modified stuttering techniques, try them in one or two of your least feared situations. When you have successful experiences in them move on to a slightly more feared situation, and so on. This gives you a guide to progress in self-therapy.

Above all, keep in mind that the less you struggle in your efforts not to stutter, and the less you avoid feared words and situations, the less you will stutter in the long run. You do not become fluent by fighting desperately to be fluent. This is what stutterers spend a great deal of time and energy doing, and this is probably the biggest reason why they continue to stutter. In this sense, fluency comes in the back door. It is a by-product of your really not caring whether you are fluent or not. You will steadily improve in the desired ways as you carry out your new speech behaviors in more and more situations, so they become increasingly automatic and integrated into your day-to-day living.

It's not a matter of luck. You make your own "luck." You can get there!

From One Stutterer To Another

SPENCER F. BROWN

We stutterers all know the feeling of panic of a tough block. To some of us this feeling is frequent and painfully familiar. At such moments the thing to do, hard as it may be, is to cool it. I have found that it helps to remember the words of a collect from the Episcopal Book of Common Prayer: "O Lord . . . who hast safely brought us to the beginning of this day."

In other words, you've come this far, you've come to *this* stuttering moment. You have survived all your former troubles including your speech problem. You've been in all sorts of agonizing situations before, and you've managed to get through them. At a moment of near panic you can't be expected to tell yourself at length what I've just been saying, but you can compress it into thinking, "I'm still here. Cool it!"

Besides telling yourself this, what do you do to handle a terribly tense block and the seeming impossibility of uttering the word you're trying to speak? First, stop trying to say the word. Then immediately try to ease it out. This is a technique taught by some of the most effective speech therapists. It would seem to be an obvious way of dealing with those ghastly blocks, yet few stutterers seem to discover this technique by themselves.

I'm now going to make a suggestion that will bring me angry letters from some speech pathologists and even, perhaps, from some stutterers. I suggest that you follow what is the almost universal practice of stutterers and on occasion use an easy word in place of a hard one. When you're having a particularly difficult time I see nothing wrong with this common practice of word substitution. I am well aware of the theory that holds that substitution of easy words for feared words increases the stutterer's fear of nonfluency. It is said that if you don't meet head-on the challenge of the fear of stuttering on a certain word, your fear of that word, and of stuttering in general, will increase. This is supposed to increase and perpetuate your problem. I'll admit that this reasoning makes good sense, but I know of no clear scientific proof of the theory.

Theory aside, the fact remains that only with expert clinical guidance can a stutterer learn to avoid substitution on a day after day, month after month basis in all speaking situations.

Furthermore, in my acquaintance with speech pathologists who are themselves stutterers, I have detected substitutions in the speech of each one. Although not frequently, those people whose clinical theories condemn substitution sometimes use substitutions themselves. Why not make life a bit easier for yourself once in a while? Don't make a habit of substitution, but don't feel guilty about using it now and then.

We stutterers have to learn to accept with as much tranquility as we can the fact that we stutter. This is not the same thing as "being resigned to it." Passive resignation never helped anyone. This resigned attitude implies an over-valuation of the importance of fluency. You don't resign yourself to having a hang-nail. You resign yourself only to something you regard as a great misfortune. If you think fluency of speech is the most important thing in life, maybe you should reconsider your priorities. One of the most successful and widely loved men of our era was Eisenhower. During press conferences he was hesitant, repetitive, and often failed to make sense. Many of his interruptions were exactly like those disfluencies people call stuttering. The important difference is that Ike wasn't distressed by his non-fluent speech. We can learn to overlook our own disfluency. Sometimes my wife will say to me, "You're stuttering a lot today." Often I'll reply that I wasn't aware of it. I'm happy when this occurs, for it indicates that I am more interested in the person I'm talking with and what I'm saying than in whether or not I'm being fluent.

If you're not able to find a speech therapist to help you, other kinds of people can often be of great assistance. My high school chemistry teacher, a former stutterer, gave up his lunch hour twice a week to talk with me about my speech. He didn't pretend to be a therapist. Since he didn't know exactly how he had gotten over his stuttering, he wisely refrained from making any specific suggestions. Rather, he listened and occasionally asked questions that helped me analyze what I was doing. My stuttering didn't cease, but I felt a lot less concerned about it and much better about myself.

Perhaps you can find this kind of sympathetic friend who will listen while you talk about your stuttering. Let him know you don't expect advice. You don't expect him to be a clinician, just a friend. I shouldn't say "just," for this sort of friend is priceless and hard to find. If you know another stutterer probably both of you can profit from talking about speech problems, provided you don't try to give each other advice.

Don't expect that psychotherapy will help your stuttering much. A psychiatrist or psychologist is trained to deal with emotional and neurotic problems. If you have severe emotional problems, by all means get the sort of help a psychiatrist or psychologist is trained to give you; but remember, "nervousness" is common to all people. Don't expect him to improve your stuttering appreciably. Learning how to deal with your other problems will doubtless make life easier, and sometimes this has an indirect effect on stuttering. But, beware the well-intentioned amateur who thinks he can "help" even though he has no training.

So you're cut off from qualified professional help? Well, you've got plenty of company! Most of the other people in the world who need any given type of specialized help, such as speech therapy, counseling, medical or dental care, never get it either. But somehow they mostly manage to make do. Professional therapy is great, but if you can't get it, don't bewail its absence. After all, fellow stutterers, there are strengths and resources within each of us. Only through these can we ever really accomplish anything.

Reducing The Fear of Stuttering

WILLIAM D. TROTTER

In order to reduce the amount of stuttering you do you must reduce your fear of stuttering. One way of reducing your fear is by increasing the amount of speaking you do, particularly in situations that you customarily avoid. The more speaking you do the more you will find out that stuttering isn't as fearful as you think. In general, the penalties attached to stuttering are not as great as you might imagine them to be.

You can get a good estimate of your speaking time by keeping a *speaking time record*. Carry a small notebook with you and two or three times a day jot down the persons with whom you have spoken and the approximate amount of time in minutes and seconds that you spoke to them. With a little practice it is relatively easy to estimate the amount of time you have spent talking with a person. At the end of the day just add up your total amount of talking time. Although there are wide individual differences, the average speaking time of a person who stutters is about 24 minutes; the average for a person who does not stutter is 44 minutes. It would probably be a good idea if you tried to speak as much as the average person. In general the amount of improvement you make will depend on the amount of talking you do, especially if you do this talking in situations you ordinarily avoid. In order to determine what kinds of speaking situations you avoid, keep a *speaking time record* for a week and classify situations such as talking to strangers in face-to-face speaking situations, talking to friends or acquaintances in face-to-face speaking situations, telephone calls to strangers, telephone calls to friends or acquaintances, speaking in discussion groups, speaking in class, and speaking to a member of the family, etc.

If you find that you customarily avoid the telephone, as many stutterers do, you will find it helpful to make some telephone calls every day. One way of getting over a fear is by doing the thing you're afraid of and finding out it is not as fearful as you had anticipated. Maybe you will find this record helpful to you.

Another way of helping yourself with your stuttering is to read while looking into a mirror. You do this in a place where you can be heard by at least one person, otherwise you probably won't stutter. After you have looked at yourself stuttering in the mirror for several hours your stuttering will be less frightening to you; this seems to carry over into your everyday speaking. Watching yourself stutter in a mirror makes you more objective and less emotional about your stuttering. Try to do this mirror work for at least fifteen minutes a day.

Listening to yourself stutter on a tape recorder is another good way of helping reduce your fear of stuttering. You should time your stuttering blocks and count the number of times you stutter. You will probably find that your blocks are not as long as you thought they were and that you actually stuttered about half as much as you expected you would. Learn to be more realistic! By listening to yourself stutter you accustom yourself to the sound of stuttering; when you are in a real speaking situation and you hear yourself stutter you're not as likely to panic.

You will feel better about your speech if you reduce the number of times you substitute non-feared words for feared ones. To test this out make five telephone calls and keep an account of the number of times you substituted non-feared words for feared ones. Then make five more telephone calls in which you try to make as few substitutions as possible. You should feel better about your speech when you are not substituting words or switching phrases to avoid stuttering You may find that your fear of stuttering is actually *more* of a problem than your stuttering.

Stuttering on purpose or "faking" at the beginning of a conversation might help you stutter less severely and less frequently throughout the rest of the conversation. To see if this idea is of any help to you fake some stuttering (any kind of stuttering may be used as long as it is clearly recognizable to the listener as stuttering) in ten conversations. Try ten more conversations without faking. See if there is a reduction in the frequency and severity of your stuttering when you faked stuttering at the beginning of the conversation. You might find that when you do this imitation stuttering you rarely experience real stuttering. This is because when you stutter on purpose you will feel little or no tendency to be anxious about whether you are going to stutter. When you go ahead and stutter on purpose you're not apt to become as tense or bothered about whether or not you're going to stutter. At first you may not be very successful in stuttering on purpose in more difficult speaking situations; gradually, you might become more successful in those where you ordinarily stutter severely.

Most people are somewhat tense talking to stutterers because they do not know how to react. Perhaps they believe that the stutterer is very sensitive about his problem and are afraid they will say or do something that will hurt his feelings. One way to make your listener feel at ease about your stuttering is to tell an occasional joke about it. If you are in a bad block and just can't get a word out you might say, "Well, if I don't get this word out soon we might be here all night." It's a good idea to have a healthy sense of humor about your stuttering. You might try one or two of these jokes on your friends to see if it puts them a little more at ease when talking to you.

Sometimes it is helpful to explain something about your stuttering to people who are important to you. This person might be a parent, teacher, friend, employer or a fellow worker. You might explain, for example, how you would like to be treated by your listener when you are stuttering. The purpose of this is to make you and the people you speak with more relaxed concerning your stuttering. If you feel that a person understands your stuttering you are likely to stutter less to that person. An open and honest attitude is healthy for all people involved.

You might find it helpful to adopt a more simple way of stuttering. This could consist of an easy prolongation of the first sound or syllable of the word. Listen to your own recording of this on tape and watch your performance of it in the mirror. After you have arrived at the point where you are adept and at ease using this pattern of stuttering on the tape recorder you should introduce it into your easier speaking situations; later, introduce it gradually into your more difficult speaking situations.

During the past twenty-five years there has been much interest in the effect of masking noise on stuttering. For two and a half years I used a portable masking noise generator. Whenever I felt I would stutter or was in the middle of a stuttering block I would turn the generator on and instantly hear a 90 to 100dB low frequency masking noise in my ears. I used this aid in all types of speaking situations, especially those in which I had most difficulty such as telephoning or giving a lecture. When I used the aid I had about one-fourth the number of stutterings and only an occasional one would be longer than one second in length. Although there was a reduction in both the frequency and duration of stuttering, the stuttering was never entirely eliminated. Whether or not such a device would help you would be difficult to predict.

I have also used an instrument that delivers a masking noise whenever you speak. This instrument is turned on automatically by the sound of the voice by a microphone attached to your throat. Or, you might find an electronic metronome useful; the beat of the metronome is fed into the ears through a cord from a small container carried in the pocket.

If you are like most stutterers you will probably not be too enthusiastic about using any of these electronic devices to help your stuttering. Although I have tried these instruments with a great number of stutterers, I have never found a stutterer who would wear one for anything but a short period of time. Perhaps the reluctance to use such aids is regarded as a sign of weakness. I do not think you should buy an electronic aid until you have had a chance to try it for several weeks. Neverthless, research has shown that such devices do improve fluency. As fluency improves the fear of stuttering decreases and as the fear decreases the fluency improves still further.

Several novels feature stutterers in important character roles. It would be valuable for you to read these books because after reading them you will have to conclude that a stutterer can be respected despite his stuttering. Respect, I think, is what the stutterer most longs for and finds hard to obtain because of his speech. In *Two Hours on Sunday* by Joseph Pillitteri one of the three or four principal characters is McHaney, a professional football coach and a stutterer. Brian Moore's *The Revolution Script* features as a kidnapper a stutterer known as C.T. (Jacques Cosette-Trudel). One of the two principal characters in Joseph Hayes novel *Like Any Other Fugitive* is Laurel Taggart, a girl stutterer who is on the run from her father. Herman Wouk's novel *The Winds of War* describes a fictional meeting between Somerset Maugham, the English author and stutterer, and President Roosevelt during World War II.

Advice To People Who Stutter

JOHN L. BOLAND, JR.

Stuttering in children can often be relieved through counseling and psychotherapy in working with the child and his parents, but as you probably already are aware, nobody knows how to 'cure' stuttering in adolescents and adults. However, you can work with your speech difficulties so as to help yourself feel less victimized by your stuttering.

It is important that you learn as much as possible about how you stutter and what you do when you stutter so that you can modify your symptoms in ways described by VanRiper, Sheehan and others. This knowledge of symptom modification techniques should help. It is possible, however, to worry too much about symptoms and ways of controlling them. Stutterers are usually too inhibited already and symptom modification procedures can be another kind of inhibition. Symptom controls, at best, are an uncertain aid and the stutterer should be aware that they are not sure and certain answers to his problem.

Stutterers come in all sizes and shapes but most of the stutterers I have known have characteristic personality problems. Most are perfectionistic. They tend to be too guilty—too anxious —too worried—too indecisive—and too inhibited. They have trouble getting along with themselves comfortably and working effectively with other people.

Most stutterers have trouble enjoying themselves. They tend to visualize themselves as always competing with other people trying to decide who is best on one ladder or another. They are engaged in a long-term 'identity crisis.' They would have these personality difficulties even if their stuttering symptoms were somehow miraculously removed.

You can learn something about your particular symptoms and you can modify them. However, in my opinion, your biggest struggle will be involved with changing your personality problems. You need to communicate more openly and easily with other people including being frank about your stuttering. You need to be warmer and more loving, to be more spontaneous and flexible, to be a more truly 'human' being. These are worthwhile goals for everybody but particularly for a stutterer.

You should start right away working on these problems with

71

someone who is knowledgeable about stuttering and is a competent psychotherapist. He may be a speech pathologist, a psychiatrist, a psychologist or possibly a social worker. Most all stutterers need to continuously work on changing their outlook on life—a lifetime goal.

Message To Adult Stutterers

GERALD R. MOSES

As a person who has stuttered for some time you have probably been more preoccupied and perplexed about this troublesome problem than any other aspect of your life. You have found that your stuttering interferes with and complicates even the most basic relationships with other people. Your expectations and hopes for personal, social and professional success have been limited by your feelings of being an inadequate talker.

You have found that concern for what others think of you has made you feel trapped and frustrated. You have wondered why you can talk freely in one situation and not at all in another. Most of all, you have asked, "Why me? Why do I stutter and my friends do not?" You have tried to follow suggestions given by others. "Slow down, think what you are going to say, whistle, etc." You have even invented some of your own techniques for preventing the occurrence of stuttering. Most of these suggestions have had some foundation in distracting your attention from stuttering. Some of them have even worked for awhile. But temporary relief due to distraction has not solved your difficulties.

You have found much of what you have read and heard about stuttering to be confusing and embarrassing. While some writers feel that you stutter because you are physically different from people who do not stutter, others seem convinced that your stuttering lies in an emotional problem. Actually, persons who stutter seem to fall within the same range of physical and emotional characteristics as persons who do not stutter. The real difference between those who stutter and those who do not seems to be that stutterers stutter.

As the problem of stuttering develops, easy repetitions and prolongations are replaced by struggled attempts to say words. Embarrassment and the avoidance of words, situations and certain listeners occurs and a degree of emotionality is injected which complicates and compounds the problem. Penalty reactions by listeners convince you that your speech is unpleasant. This leads to further desperate attempts to prevent the occurrence of stuttering by whatever means available; struggle and avoidance are among the most commonly used.

During periods of crisis or conflict alternative ways to cope with and resolve problems present themselves. The range of alternatives is extreme. On the one hand we find flight or avoidance. On the other hand we find fight or struggle. Depending on the occasion either extreme might be appropriate, but a reasonable compromise seems to be more healthy, more effective and more generally used. When extreme measures become the rule the original problem has been compounded. On one hand, the problem becomes a struggle problem; on the other, an avoidance problem. The problem of stuttering develops or worsens when extreme reactions become learned as routine responses to what was once a more simple problem of speech disfluency.

Crucial to this point is the fact that struggle and avoidance *worsen* a problem of stuttering. Easy repetitions of sounds become hard repetitions with tension and facial contortion when force and hurry are added to them. Audiences react negatively to the struggle, and this convinces you that you must "try harder" so you increase your struggle. Similarly, penalty reactions to your stuttering prompt you to avoid or conceal your stuttering. Your speech becomes cautious and backward-moving. Your attention is directed to planning escape from stuttered words rather than to planning your thoughts. Avoidance strengthens your need to be fluent. The most evil part of this development is the subtle way in which struggle and avoidance become a part of you. They become involuntary and you do not recognize when you use them.

If you are serious about working to resolve your stuttering problem then it is time to change your approach to the problem. Easy ways out of difficulty are momentarily convenient, but in the long run they reinforce the problem. Although a step-by-step approach to solving a problem of stuttering does not account for individual differences among those who stutter, the following suggestions are placed in the order of their importance.

Reduce Avoidances. Determine to reduce your use of avoidances. Try to stutter openly and audibly. Let your stutterings be heard and seen rather than continue to conceal them by hurry and quiet. Try to keep your stuttering forward-moving and purposeful rather than postponed and half-hearted. Try to maintain eye contact with your listeners. Looking away severs the communication link with your audience and convinces them that you are ashamed and disgusted with the way that you talk. When you present yourself in an embarrassed and uncomfortable way you are more likely to receive negative audience reactions than if you stutter openly and severely. Deliberately enter previously feared situations. Judge your performance on the basis of the degree to which you approached the situation rather than on the basis of how much you stuttered or how fluent you were. Begin to recognize yourself as you are and as you want to be rather than as you think others want you to be. All of us need to be loved by, and in close contact with, other people. However, too much "human respect" makes us prisoners of what we think others want us to be.

Stutter in an Easier Way.   When you are openly tackling the majority of your moments of stuttering you can try to change their form. Look at your stutterings objectively rather than emotionally. Study them by holding on to them longer than it would have taken to stutter-out the troublesome word. Resist the impulse to get the stuttering over with quickly. Although it is difficult to become less emotional about what you do, you need to become more realistic about yourself. For awhile, you must place greater emphasis on recognizing how you talk rather than on what others think of you.

Experiment with different ways to stutter for the purpose of learning how you stutter and the strength of your stuttering. Recognize and specify what you do when you stutter. Begin by listing the struggle behaviors that you use which are not a part of the act of speaking. Become aware of head or arm movements, eye blinking, other movements or body rigidity, lip-smacking or other noises, puffing of the cheeks or pursing of the lips. You will seek to eliminate these behaviors by increasing your awareness of them and separating them from your attempts to talk. Practice their use and insert them voluntarily into your speech when you have moments of less stuttering. Show yourself that they are not required for talking by using them independently of real and severe moments of stuttering.

Other behaviors which characterize your stuttering can be changed and normalized. Make an inventory of speech related struggle that accompanies your stuttering. Factors such as hurrying the utterance, tension in the lips, face and throat, and unusual preformations of sounds should be noted.

Normalize your attempts to say stuttered words. Normal speech is easy and forward-moving. Movements are released effortlessly. Try to prolong the first sound in a troublesome word until you feel you can release the rest of the word easily. If prolongations are uncomfortable for you, try an easy repetition of the first *syllable* of the word. Maintain the prolongation or repetition *out loud*. Make your approach to the word purposeful and straightforward. Your task is to learn to approach your stutterings openly and honestly and to eliminate the effort and hurry associated with previous attempts to talk. Judge your performance based on the degree of approach (stutter loud enough and long enough to examine what you are doing) and the degree of ease of release.

This is strong medicine! It is contrary to what you have improvised and learned. The emphasis is upon controlled *exhibition* of your stuttering, not upon inhibition. The number of times that you have previously inhibited your stuttering should suggest that many exhibitions will be needed to change significantly your manner of talking. Comfort in the use of normalized stuttering will follow only after much exercise. You may wish to select a friend or confidant with whom you can discuss your successes and failures, your heroics and flops. Your goal is not perfect speech, but rather the reduction of concern about your speech and the normalization of your attempts to talk.

Recognize and Tolerate Normal Disfluency. Normal speech contains disfluencies of many types. Easy repetitions of words and phrases, revisions, and incomplete phrases are a few types of normal disfluency. When these occur, and as long as they are *not* used as avoidance devices, they should be recognized as normal and not as symptoms of stuttering. Intolerance of normal disfluency causes you to try to talk with perfect fluency, an unattainable goal for anyone. Listen to these breaks in fluency in the speech of nonstuttering talkers. When the same kind of disfluencies occur in your own speech, they should be accepted and viewed as normal.

Again, these suggestions are strong medicine. I appreciate how difficult they seem. I encourage you to give them a fair trial. Finally, accept my best wishes for success and my respect for your determination to approach and resolve your problem of stuttering.

No Stutterer Is An Island Unto Himself

Gary N. LaPorte

When are you going to start doing what you are supposed to be doing? This question, like many others, is asked and the usual reply is, "I'm trying but I just don't seem to be getting anywhere." "Why?" To examine some of the common things that stutterers use to help themselves several stutterers were asked for a brief list of things they use. Perhaps some of the things they use to help themselves are things which you have used. If so, ask yourself the question, "Have they given me long lasting relief from stuttering, or merely temporary relief?" Here is the list: (1) Substituting another word for the word I feel I will stutter on, (2) using the syllable "uh" to get through a word, (3) laughing to get the word started, (4) talking slowly, or with a ryhthmical pattern of speech, (5) snapping my fingers to get the word started, (6) stopping and attempting to start over again, and (7) counting on someone else to say the word for me.

These devices, tricks or whatever you wish to call them are but a few of the many ingenious ways that stutterers have discovered to combat their day to day fight with communicative difficulty. Are they useful, or are they useful only temporarily?

We should realize that these tricks serve two purposes; to either prevent, or to get through, a feared word. Most stutterers feel they need some ways to cope with their stuttering, but these may not be as helpful in the long run as they first appear to be.

Unfortunately, these devices all serve to help maintain the problem of stuttering and result in the avoidance rather than the confrontation of stuttering. Avoidance can be defined as a process of shying away from the responsibility of facing your problem. You may say to yourself, "I do stutter, I know I do, so I am facing it." This is not true because although you recognize you stutter, you still continue to try to hide it. Facing your stuttering means (1) Saying 'I stutter' and discussing it openly with as many people as you can, (2) Learning some more positive ways of assisting yourself through your moments of stuttering every day. (3) Giving up your old tricks, and (4) Admitting to yourself that your stuttering presents a real problem. The following suggestions may help you to work on your stuttering.

What should you talk about when you discuss your stuttering? Whenever you have an opportunity to discuss your stuttering with someone, do it! Talk about such things as their feelings toward someone who stutters or the things you have done in the past to hide your own stuttering. Discuss why you have tried to hide your stuttering and the problems you have had finding a job. This will be difficult for you to do, I know, because I experienced this myself. But after forcing myself to do this many times it became easier and well worth the effort. The more frank you become about your stuttering the more you will enjoy talking about it and the less you will try to hide it.

What can you do to make your stuttering come out easier, and with less tension and struggle? Deliberately stutter! Yes, stutter on purpose in as many situations as possible, but stutter in a different way. Use a bounce and repeat the first syllable one, two or three times in this manner: "ta-tent" or "Da-Da-Diane" or "ska-ska-ska-school." Use the short "a" vowel because this is usually unlike the real vowel that goes with the word; it is easier to go from a syllable that has a vowel unlike the first vowel in the word. For words which have a short "a" like "car" maintain this short "a" because switching to another vowel would sound awkward.

What should you do when you find yourself stuttering on a word? Don't hide your stuttering. Instead stutter obviously. Stop what you are saying and say that same word over and over again before you continue. If you have difficulty saying it again use the bounce pattern. It may sound like stuttering, but it will be easier stuttering with a lot less frustration. For example, suppose you stuttered on the word 'tomorrow' in the sentence, "I'll call you tomorrow." Stop after 'tomorrow' then say 'tomorrow' over by bouncing and then continue the rest of the sentence. Face your problem, don't hide it. With practice, this will help you stutter more easily and with less frustration.

What should you do if you feel you will stutter on a word? Say to yourself, "I am going to say that word even though I may stutter on it, but I'm going to say it with a bounce." Or you might want to prolong the first sound in much the same way you would hold onto a note if singing. If you can say the word fluently, this is fine, but I would advise you to use some deliberate form of stuttering as noted above. Otherwise, you may become too sure of yourself and have a tendency to use fluent speech too soon. This might result in more stuttering at first because you have no means for dealing with your blocks. Later you can use more fluency if you like.

What can you do when you are stuck on a word? Concentrate on the *next* sound in the word and then go on to that sound, and then to the next sound, and so on until you have moved progressively through the word. For example, if you're stuck on the "b" in birthday, concentrate on the next sound "ir" and then "th," "d," and "ay" thus moving through the word. If you prefer, you can also stop after you have moved through the word and say it over again using one of the bounce patterns.

These suggestions for helping you face your stuttering by discussing it openly with other people and by deliberately stuttering in an easier manner will show that you are not afraid to stutter and can stutter in front of other people in any situation.

Perhaps all of these suggestions have interested you, and you might even try one or two of them. Merely trying, however, will not be enough. You will have to make yourself do these things and this will not be easy. You will need much courage. All I can say is that these suggestions helped me, and I feel they will help you. If you are willing to take responsibility and put these suggestions into practice, then you may find you need to modify them to fit into the work schedule you have determined for yourself. Be careful, however, not to modify them to the point where they cause you to go back to your former habits of avoiding. Always keep the idea of facing your stuttering foremost in your mind; do not avoid.

"No Stutterer is an Island Unto Himself." You must come to the realization that you must communicate with people as much as you can. You must not hide your stuttering, but bring it out into the open and work on it.

Finally, a speech pathologist can be of assistance and should be consulted if at all possible. He may be able to provide advice and suggestions that will help you deal with your communication difficulties.

A Therapy Experience

HUGO H. GREGORY

The story of my stuttering therapy that I would like to tell here began when I was fifteen years old. Fortunately, I like to browse through periodicals, and one day while doing so I read about an institution 1500 miles away from my home in Arkansas that offered help for stutterers. At this center I was shown that I could modify my stuttering by prolonging vowel sounds and making lighter consonant contacts. This approach brought great relief and hope that I might, after all, aspire to become a lawyer and take part in politics. This method seemed to be "the way" to break the habit of stuttering.

Although I was conscientious and practiced using my manual of words and sentences beginning with all the vowels and consonants, a few months after I returned home I began to slip; the vicious circle of increased fear and stuttering began to return. However, I never again struggled as much with my speech as I had before this initial therapy.

I returned to the program the following year and began to learn some of the important lessons that have helped me to speak with increased freedom and versatility each year. I had previously focused too much on "controlling" my stuttering and had been willing to do anything (prolong the vowel, or use "light contacts") to keep from stuttering. I began to realize that I was concentrating too much on the *speech* aspect of therapy and was missing the part which had to do with *attitude*. I recall that the clinicians had talked about the way in which stutterers, in fact all people tend to overemphasize what they perceive as a problem. Stutterers tend to become very sensitive about the fluency of their speech. This is easy to understand, but it is not easy to change! As I examined my attitude I began to see that if I stuttered in a situation I was very hard on myself and considered myself pretty much a failure. Later on, after I was in college, Wendell Johnson's ideas helped me to understand that I should not attempt to evaluate myself as "either-or," (*either* I am a stutterer *or* I am not a stutterer.) I began to view myself as a person who sometimes stuttered as I talked and that I was going through a process of changing. This process involved evaluating what happened when I stuttered, modifying the way I talked, evaluating again, changing again, etc. It also involved changing my attitude of wanting to "beat" stuttering rather than studying it and changing it. It helped me learn that others did not think about my stuttering nearly as much as I did.

During my first two years in college I began to see more clearly that a stutterer has to take responsibility for making others feel comfortable in his presence. If he can be less sensitive about his stuttering those around him will be more comfortable, this will make him more at ease, he will stutter less, and so it goes; the vicious circle will be put into reverse. Since I was doing something constructive about my speech, I could smile about difficulty more. I could even feign some voluntary disfluency. The writings of Van Riper influenced me to be willing to *stutter on purpose*. I have always been fascinated by the idea of experimenting with all of the obvious or subtle ways I can be disfluent. In addition to studying what occurs when I speak that, as Williams puts it, interferes with the flow of speech and learning to change that pattern, I made a game of playing with my speech pattern, "do-do-ing th-i-i-is or tha-a-t." In this way the fear of speaking has melted away. I can speak differently, and of course I can communicate better, but it has been very important to me to be willing to be disfluent voluntarily. For me, this counteracts the rather deeply ingrained desire to be perfectly fluent and keeps the fear "doused."

Between the ages of fifteen and twenty I worked rather intensely on my speech and gradually realized that I would need to work on situations of increasing difficulty by planning, experiencing and then planning again, etc., until I became more and more confident. For example, during my freshman year in college I worked on introducing myself. After working to keep eye contact with my listener, I worked on modifying my speech and using some voluntary disfluency when saying "I'm Hugo Gre-Gregory." By the end of the year I never avoided introducing myself or making introductions.

Another general philosophy of my therapy has been that by tackling situations of greater difficulty, others which were once hard become easier. Thus, in my junior year in college I felt ready for public speaking. Sure, I stuttered when making a speech, but conversations with one or two people became much easier. Eventually getting up to speak before a group became easier, too!

At about this time I began my training as a speech pathologist and embarked upon a career, as my wife and children tell friends, of being a "professional stutterer." By the way, I've always noticed that when my wife tells some person "Hugo is a professional stutterer," the person looks somewhat perplexed as if to say, "Does he stutter?" or, "Why do you mention it?" The point is that we are very open about my stuttering. I found out very early that this attitude is an important ingredient in therapy.

Do not get the impression that I am advocating being anything but realistic about stuttering. Apprehension about saying certain words and the dread of stuttering in a situation are very real social and vocational handicaps for a stutterer. I know it has been easier for me as a stutterer during my adult years to be in speech pathology and to be working with stutterers. Coping with a fear-associated problem such as stuttering is difficult. Still, when we have such a problem we have to enter into activities, preferably with the help of a speech pathologist, that enable us to make realistic change and improvements. Reducing the fear and increasing the comfort when communicating can be very rewarding!

I also found, in working on my speech, that one makes many discoveries that can be applied advantageously to daily living. From the time I began therapy I have realized that I must take responsibility for my behavior and the way in which others evaluate me. In addition, I became aware of the tendency to lean on my stuttering as an excuse for not participating in some activity or for not being as successful as I might strive to be.

I continue to learn. I have practiced relaxation procedures as one approach to modifying the muscular tension involved in stuttering and to diminishing emotional arousal during speaking. Relaxation has been generally useful when I have needed to be more calm during a crisis.

As a speech pathologist working with adult stutterers I have found that the most important factors that determine progress are (1) that the stutterer have a goal that requires better speech, and (2) that he form the habit of working consistently and steadily to accomplish his purpose. Someone once told me that the price of better speech is keeping steadily at it. Many stutterers can have a speech pathologist to help them evaluate their problem and guide them in therapy. To those who cannot have this help in therapy I say "Find out whatever you can whenever you can, and then work steadily." At the end of every week, those having therapy and those not having therapy should ask as I always have, "What have I learned about my speech this week?"

Four Steps to Freedom

RICHARD M. BOEHMLER

As an adult seeking advice for your stuttering it seems to me four basic problems must be solved:

A. *Identifying* the specific nature of your stuttering,

B. *Developing* an effective therapy program,

C. *Successfully carrying* out the therapy program,

D. *Maintaining* success in the future.

Now these four problems can be solved. Stuttering is not the mysterious dilemma it was years ago. Although the nature of stuttering varies from individual to individual, it can be understood. Effective treatment methods have been developed, but to be effective the treatment must be appropriate to *your* specific stuttering pattern. The first step is to *identify* yourself.

A. Knowing that you "stutter" is not enough. If it were, advice for treatment would be much simpler. However, your stuttering is probably not the same as mine was, did not have the same causal history, and would not necessarily respond to the same treatment. Your stuttering is unique to you and its uniqueness must be identified.

Self diagnosis is a difficult task at best, so you may need professional help. If help is not available there is a great deal you can do on your own. You can start by describing exactly what you do or do not do when you wish to speak. Be as specific as you can. Describe specific movements, feelings and actions. If the speech production mechanism is blocked, describe exactly which muscles do not move in the appropriate fashion. Describe ways in which your communication patterns differ from those of your friends, or from your own patterns when you are communicating freely and successfully. It would be helpful to divide your observations into five categories:

1. *Involuntary Fluency Breakdowns:* Breaks in the flow of speech which you did not intentionally produce and which you find undesirable;

2. *Interfering Hypertension:* Specific muscle tensions which make speaking difficult. For example, tensions in your arms do not effect speech production, but excessive vocal cord tension would if this tension interfered with vibrations;

3. *Speech Patterns Used to Avoid:* Breakdowns such as deliberately starting over, using a pause, talking slowly, and substituting a word synonym when a breakdown has occurred or is anticipated;

4. *Patterns Used to Cope with a Breakdown:* Speech and non-speech behaviors used after the flow of speech has stopped such as increased air pressure against the "blocked" articulatory position (forcing the lips apart), or releasing the "block" by increased tension in non-speech muscles (foot stomping), or relaxing the muscles involved in the "block," etc.;

5. *Self-Concept as a Communicator:* Thinking of how you will speak rather than what you will say, or remembering "stuttering" as the highlight of the conversation and imagining yourself a speaking failure, etc.

An unlimited number of examples of questions would need to be presented to cover all potential patterns of communication covered by "stuttering." Chapters 6 and 7 in Van Riper's *The Nature of Stuttering* would provide helpful background reading for increasing your ability to do this step well.

Two words of caution! First, a perfect flow of language formulation and speech production is a rare skill. Most of us have errors in formulation and imperfections in our speech production. Include these in your analysis but be sure to distinguish between those patterns, including breakdowns, which are acceptable and those which are not. Compare what you do against what your friends do. They also repeat sounds, words and phrases, interject "uh" or stop while saying a difficult word. Therapy should lead toward acceptable, free flowing speech but not *perfect fluency.* Second, objectivity is a serious problem in self-analysis. In the absence of a speech clinician to aid you, ask your spouse, friend or teacher to point out what they see and hear you do as you communicate. This will aid you in obtaining specific descriptions of your stuttering. The use of a tape recorder will also help.

If a clinician were to make the above analysis I would expect him to spend several hours in most cases. Expect no less and even more from yourself. A thorough job of self-identification is critical to proceeding or moving ahead successfully.

B. Many therapies have been developed to deal with "stuttering." The ideas presented by other contributors to this booklet include many of the possibilities and are quite adequate for dealing with most advanced stuttering behaviors; restatements and extensions of these points are not necessary. Your task is to select those ideas which most closely fit *your specific* problem.

Breakdowns from *excess tension* may reflect an inappropriate articulation rate, poor formulation of thoughts, anxieties about blocking, anxieties about speaking situations, or more general anxieties about yourself. A clear understanding of the nature of stuttering can lead directly to the appropriate therapy. Common sense, past experiences with therapy and reading the suggestions of various authors may be adequate for you to proceed at this point, but professional help may be needed in selecting the appropriate therapy.

One note of caution. None of us, whether stutterer or clinician, can be 100% correct. Our diagnosis of ourself or of others is subject to error. Selection of the appropriate therapy is based on our most educated opinion after careful study. Likewise, in diagnosing your own problem, don't hesitate to evaluate the effectiveness of the therapy if it is not helpful. Continuing ineffective therapy is not only expensive but a waste of precious time. Select what seems to be the most appropriate therapy and put it into practice. If it doesn't work within a reasonable time, try to evaluate why and then change it accordingly.

C. Making a therapy program successful involves a great deal more than correct identification of the problem and the selection of appropriate therapy. It requires consistent, devoted and thorough application of the therapy program. Whether you are working by yourself or with the aid of a speech clinician, the success of therapy is primarily up to you. This is not a cop-out on my part. No one but myself improved my speech. Others have helped me by providing information, giving emotional support, identifying bias, etc., but the dirty work of therapy is, and always has been, *my* responsibility. Likewise, I have not changed the communication skills of any of my clients. I have only helped them to help themselves. They did the job if the job was done. Even in other helping professions the clinician only helps; he does not do the basic job. Your body heals itself, the surgeon only helps the process. Just as the body cells must do the major part in healing a wound, you must do the major part in changing behavior patterns, in developing communication skills, and in obtaining freedom to communicate. Many failures are due to the individual spending too *small* a portion of his talking time learning new ways of behaving, and too *large* a portion of his communication time practicing old patterns. This just doesn't work! Therapy must be practiced full time to be highly successful. You must feel that you are on the right track and you must be committed to putting the program into practice. Plan your work well, then work your plan harder than you have ever worked before. Success will follow.

D. Relapses into old stuttering patterns are the rule, not the exception. Follow through: provide for maintenance and reinforcement of success. Whether the changes you make involve your self-image, decreasing blocks, coping better with blocks, more fluent speech, or greater freedom to communicate, the change will not maintain itself. Patterns of life which have been established and maintained for many years cannot be changed in a few months and then continued spontaneously on their own. Therapy must be continued until new patterns are as automatic and as much a part of you as was your old stuttering. Not continuing to maintain the results of your therapy program will not only make a relapse practically inevitable, but will also require some degree of starting over and going over the same ground again to bring back the success you earned. Remember how you improved, and keep the improvement going.

Stuttering is no longer the dilemma of the communication disorders. It can be changed. If freedom to communicate is not yours because of stuttering, it is my advice that you develop a very specific understanding of *your* communication patterns. Based on your understanding choose the most appropriate therapy program you can, and work at the program with more consistency, devotion and energy than any other task you've ever tackled. As success is obtained, maintain it with equal vigor. I believe that most therapy has failed because of poor diagnosis, inappropriate therapy, halfhearted application of therapy and poor follow-through. Don't make these mistakes! Identify, plan, work, and then follow-through!

Guidelines

PAUL E. CZUCHNA

By the time most stutterers become adults they have become profoundly frustrated in their efforts to speak fluently, and irritated at themselves for their failure to do so. They feel that they have at least average intelligence, but have endured endless labor and energy expended during their efforts to communicate. They feel helpless about mastering their stuttering and wonder what is wrong with them. As a result, they fear stuttering more and more and enjoy speaking less and less.

For years most adult stutterers have received well meaning suggestions that have been directly or indirectly aimed at stopping the stuttering altogether. These suggestions imply miraculously quick cures and fluent speech. "Take a deep breath before a word on which you may stutter, then say it without stuttering." "Think of what you're going to say before you say it, and you won't have any trouble," etc. You, like every other stutterer, have heard such prescriptions that imply and instill within him the belief that it is "wrong" to stutter. In his efforts to speak fluently, the stutterer becomes more and more fearful of being unable to cope with the intermittent stuttering that may occur. The more he struggles to avoid possible stuttering or attempts to hide or disguise the stuttering that cannot be avoided, the more he denies that he has a problem.

There appear to be two main types of stutterers: (1) the *covert* stutterer who attempts to avoid contacts with feared words and situations that might identify him as a possible stutterer to his listeners and (2) the *overt* stutterer who struggles laboriously through word after word as he communicates. The remaining types are varying combinations of these two. Which one are you?

Let us look at some of the communicative behavior of the *covert* stutterer and some of his associated feelings. Covert stutterers scan ahead during their utterances and continuously look for any expected word difficulty that might result in stuttering. They must be fully and constantly prepared for any emergency so they can avoid these words and not unmask themselves. When they anticipate possible stuttering they attempt to avoid direct contact with feared words. They postpone words they must say by various means until they feel they might be able to utter them more fluently. Or, at the precise moment they must utter a particular word, they use various timing devices such as eye blinks, quick body movements or gestures. Rather than endure any obvious struggle that might be interpreted as stuttering, they may attempt to get others to fill in these "key words" for them or completely give up their intent to communicate. Covert stutterers have learned which kinds of speaking situations tend to produce unavoidable stuttering and they have become masters at avoiding these situations (i.e., walking a mile or two to talk to someone rather than use the telephone; sending others on errands which involve speaking, etc.). Do you do these things?

In contrast, the more *overt* stutterer seemingly "barrels on through" words and sounds quite directly when he expects difficulty during his communication. He may not like his struggling efforts, but he has learned to endure them. At the same time he may have a minimum of word and situation avoidance since he expects to stutter anyway. He may, however, postpone word utterances and do some avoiding of his more obnoxious behaviors *during* moments of outward stuttering. These stutterers sense the penalty they receive from listeners who become impatient due to the amount of time it takes to communicate. Yet they still like to talk and do so. They resent other people filling in words for them or attempting to complete their utterances. These stutterers are often profoundly frustrated in their efforts to increase their rate of speaking, yet at the same time they exhibit many kinds of struggling behaviors that really interfere with accomplishing this. They stutter harder than they need to! They do things that actually prevent them from saying their words easily. Perhaps you do, too.

Stutterers do not need to learn how to speak fluently. They already know how to do this even though they rarely pay any attention to their fluent utterances. They may have to learn more about how to respond to the fear or experience of blocking, but they do not have to learn (as something new) to say words fluently. Some of the intense frustration comes from knowing how to say words fluently, yet finding themselves stuck and unable to do so. Stutterers need to learn what to do when they do stutter if they are to eventually reduce the fear and frustration involved. As a tentative reachable goal to shoot for, they must learn to move more easily through stuttered words rather than recoiling from them. They need other choices of ways to stutter when they expect to stutter as well as other ways of completing word utterances after they block. In short, they first need to learn a better way of stuttering, one which will interfere very little with communication. Do you know how to stutter fluently?

Most stutterers initially react with revulsion and rejection to the thought of learning to stutter differently with less struggle. After all, they have spent many years attempting either not to stutter at all, or attempting to hide stuttering when it does occur. The more *covert* stutterer may respond with extreme fear and panic even to the thought of trying to learn to stutter fluently, for he has spent considerable time and effort developing his many tricks to avoid ever being discovered as being a stutterer. The *overt* stutterer may have grave doubts that he can ever learn to stutter more effortlessly, yet recognize that this would provide some relief for him. Nevertheless, the thought of learning to stutter more fluently, as an intermediate goal to shoot for, begins eventually to become a possibility. They would prefer to have a quick cure; perhaps if they could learn to be fluent even when they do stutter, it wouldn't be so bad. How do you respond to this?

The *covert* stutterer has a longer way to go than does the more overt stutterer. The covert stutterer must first literally rediscover what he is fearful of doing by deliberately stuttering more overtly when he anticipates stuttering. To do so, he must resist using his old avoidance tricks when he expects to stutter. He must learn to endure by experiencing what he is usually only guessing he might do. The *overt* stutterer, on the other hand, must learn to examine and tolerate more and more of what he actually does when he stutters rather than deny the existence of his obvious stuttering behavior. Both overt and covert stutterers must come to know vividly what is to be changed and get a fairly clear picture of the procedures that will create a more fluent kind of stuttering. They must then learn to build solid bridges to fluency rather than repeatedly trying to jump to fluency and falling and failing. Do you know how to get out of the mess where you now are?

The following crucial experiences, which you must seek

again and again, are the basic building materials and equipment needed to build a bridge from where you are now to where you want to be in the future:

1. You are basically responsible for your own behavior, including your stuttering.
2. Stuttering can be deliberately endured, touched, maintained and studied.
3. Avoidance only increases fear and stuttering, and must be reduced.
4. Struggling, hurried escape from stuttering blockages, and recoiling away from expected or felt blockings, make stuttering worse than it need be, and tends to make it persist.
5. It is possible to release yourself voluntarily from blocking or repeating prior to completing a word utterance.
6. When a moment of stuttering occurs it can be studied, and its evil effects erased as much as possible.
7. Attending to your normal speech and adopting short, forward-moving, effortless moments of stuttering reduces more severe stuttering.
8. The self-suggestion of incoming stuttering can be resisted and words can be spoken fairly normally.
9. It is possible to build barriers to destructive listener reactions that tend to precipitate stuttering.
10. Ambivalence, anxiety, guilt and hostility can be decreased.
11. Every effort should be made to build up your ego strength, self-confidence and self-respect.
12. Society in general rewards the person who obviously confronts and attempts to deal with his stuttering.
13. It is more personally rewarding to stutter fluently than to stutter grotesquely, and it is fun to be able to talk anywhere even if you do stutter.

Will you merely read this list and then forget it? Or will you consider each item carefully and see if you can find some way to use it to help yourself?

These experiences which the stutterer must repeatedly undergo may be difficult to devise or to carry out by the stutterer alone. The stutterer feels in enough lonely isolation with his stuttering problem as it is. Therapy for stutterers ordinarily requires having a competent speech therapist available as a guide, one who can share experiences with the stutterer throughout the course of therapy. The companionship of a competent speech therapist is usually essential for therapy success. Get help if you can, but if none is available, help yourself. Others have done so!

Face Your Fears

Sol Adler

My youth, as is the case with so many stutterers, was filled with alternate hope and despair as I hungered for some relief from my stuttering. This of course is not unique; most stutterers have had similar feelings. But have you ever asked yourself what it is that really bothers you, what it is that causes despair? Is it your stuttering or is it your fear of people's reactions to your stuttering? Isn't it the latter? Most stutterers have too much anxiety about what they think people might say or might do as a result of the stuttering. These anxieties can be lessened.

I remember well these feelings of worry, anxiety, and despair. If you can learn to dissipate some of these terrible feelings—you will be able to help yourself as many other stutterers have done.

There is one effective method you can utilize to achieve this goal. Face your fears! This advice is easy to give and admittedly difficult for many of you to take; however, it is advice that has helped many stutterers and it can help you.

Learn to face your fears of stuttering in different speech situations. My involvement in such "situational-work" during my early career created peace of mind for me. It was a slow process; I didn't achieve such freedom all in one day or week or month; and it was hard work. But I did it, and others have done it, and so can you.

Somehow you must learn to desensitize yourself to the reactions of others and refuse to let people's actual or imagined responses to your stuttering continue to affect your mental health or your peace of mind.

This is easier said than done but it can be accomplished. I found that by facing my fears gradually I was able to achieve such a goal and I have known other stutterers who have "thrown" themselves into similar confrontations. Use whatever pace that best suits you but get involved, one way or another, in these confrontations with your "speech fears." There will be times when you will be unable to face the fears inherent in different situations, but persevere. Don't give up! Continue facing your fears as often as you can. Besides the peace of mind that develops, you will also become more fluent in your speech. You will find yourself manifesting lesser amounts of stuttering and that stuttering will never be as severe as it was previous to your confrontation.

You will find that as you grow older you will develop more ability to do these things. With growing maturity we can generally face our fears more frequently and more consistently. But how long do you want to wait?

List all the speech situations in which you fear stuttering. These are pretty standard situations; for example, most stutterers fear using the telephone. They experience much distress when they are called upon to answer the telephone while it rings incessantly, or conversely, when they must place a necessary call. I remember well how often I "played-deaf" when the telephone would ring. Sometimes, unfortunately, I might be standing not more than a few feet from that ringing telephone, and my protestations regarding "answer what telephone?" would be of no avail. Face this fear by making many telephone calls each day to different persons—people whose names are unknown to you. Practice stuttering while you speak to them. Stutter in different ways. For example, I once had a patient make such a call and the party on the other end turned out to be a preacher. The patient had been told he must ask for J - J - J - J but to never complete the name. The preacher was an extraordinarily kind person and evidently with some time to spare. He continually urged the patient to "take it easy" and assured him that he wouldn't hang up. For two or three minutes the patient continued repeating the initial "J" until, in sheer desperation, the preacher said, "Son, there is no "J" here. I'm sorry but I have to go," and with that he hung up. What do stutterers learn from this and similar experiences? Not to be as afraid of answering the telephone since the worst possible thing that could happen to him would be for the party to hang up on him, or to say something derogatory to him. In either case, his world doesn't end. By such experiences you will find yourself getting toughened caring less about how people might respond to you and, finally, you will be able to use the phone with lesser amounts of fear, anxiety, and stuttering.

Another classic situation most stutterers fear is asking questions of strangers. I suspect that this bothers you too. What I did, and have my patients do, is to stop people who are walking somewhere, or are in stores, and ask them questions concerning the time, directions, the price of some object, etc. All student clinicians who have trained under my supervision have been asked to do first whatever they ask the patient to accomplish. Thus they too had to first ask such questions of strangers. But since they were not stutterers they had to feign stuttering and they were required to do it very convincingly. These normal speakers discovered, as you well know, that much anxiety is experienced when asked to perform as indicated. But anxiety becomes reduced and dissipated if you engage in these kinds of situational experiences rapidly, one after another, almost without pause. For example: ask ten or fifteen people about their views regarding the cause of stuttering. You will find that after the eighth or ninth person has responded you will no longer possess all the fears you did when you initiated this exercise. Also, as a bonus, you might be surprised to find yourself actually listening to and arguing with your respondents. and actually enjoying the exercise.

To argue about and/or to discuss effectively with anyone the causes or nature of stuttering means that you have to have some relevant information about stuttering. Do you know what this speech disorder is all about? If not, you should. You should learn as much about it as is possible. If your library does not contain sufficient information, write to the editor or publisher of this booklet for additional information or, write to the American Speech and Hearing Association in Washington, D.C. for information. No longer tolerate the false information from your parents, friends, teachers or others who are interested in you, and want to help, but who are probably very ignorant about stuttering. Educate them! But educate yourself first!

I discovered also that by talking to other stutterers I received indirectly the benefits of their therapeutic experiences. Find other stutterers! It may surprise you to find out how many fellow stutterers are available. Form groups! In this way you can help each other. It will be so much easier for you when you can find someone in whom you can confide and who understands your problem. Work up your own situational assignments. Alternate as clinician and patient with the proviso that the "clinician" must first do whatever he asks the "patient" to do. Watch people closely! See how they react to your stuttering. Do you see facial grimaces or indications of shock or surprise on their faces? Occasionally you may but often you may not. You will find that when you both become objective enough to observe these people carefully, and to compare notes regarding their responses, you may even begin to enjoy the exercise. Your group should also try to obtain the services of a competent and sympathetic professional person who can guide you in discussions regarding those factors involving personality development. If not, discuss them yourselves. This kind of introspection—or self-analysis—helped me a great deal. It made me look at myself to see what made me tick. I began to realize that much of the behavior I disliked in myself was motivated by my fear of stuttering.

In summary I have suggested two matters of great importance to you regarding your stuttering: (1) Learn all about stuttering; read everything you can regarding this disorder; there is much literature available. (2) Face your fears as often and as consistently as you can. Do not give up if and when you backtrack; try to meet "head-on" these feared situations. When you can do so with some degree of consistency, you may find a new "life" awaiting you.

Some Suggestions For Adult Stutterers Who Want to Talk Easily

Dean E. Williams

For purposes of this paper, I want you to assume that I am meeting with an adult group of stutterers for the first time and that you are a member of that group. My purpose will be to suggest what I think you can do to improve the ways you talk. The major points presented in this paper are those that would be discussed and elaborated and experienced during the subsequent weeks of therapy. It is important to point out that I am talking to you as a *group;* for any one person in the group, I would direct my attention toward his own special feelings, viewpoints and needs. Because this discussion is directed toward a group, it will be necessary for each of you to think through the comments made and to apply them to your own individual problem.

. . . . . .

In working to solve a problem such as stuttering, you must first ponder the various ways that you think about the problem for they affect, in good part, what you do as you talk. They affect the observations you make, the ways you react inside, and the ways you interpret the success or failure of what you have done. Furthermore, they determine, in the main, what you will do the next time you talk.

Think about your stuttering problem. *How* do you view it? *What* do you do that you call your stuttering? *Why* do you think you do it? *What* are the most helpful things you can do when you stutter? *How* do they relate to what you believe is wrong? *What* does not help? Why? When one begins to ask questions about what he is doing, it can stimulate him to make observations about his behavior. This, in turn, encourages him to become *involved* with the ways he feels, with the ways he thinks, and with what he is doing as he talks. This is necessary! You cannot solve a problem by acting like an innocent bystander waiting for someone else to answer questions that you never thought to ask. It is *your* problem and you must face it. Perhaps I can help stimulate you to consider your own beliefs by relating examples of how a few other stutterers of different ages have viewed their stuttering. In my opinion, the ways they talk about the problem change in relation to the number of years they have attempted to cope with it.

The seven-to-nine-year-old stutterer is apt to be confused and bewildered by the ways he talks and by people's reactions to it. One second grade boy reported that when he was in kindergarten and first grade he had repeated sounds a great deal. People called it "stuttering." Now, he tensed and "pushed" to get the words out so he wouldn't "repeat," or "stutter," as he understood the meaning of the word. Now, people were calling the tensing and pushing "stuttering." He was confused!

A 9-year-old typically held his breath, blinked his eyes and tensed his jaw. This, to him, was his stuttering. One day he began taking quick breaths and then blurting the word out quickly. He reported that he was doing this so he wouldn't do the holding of breath and other behavior mentioned above. People were still reacting to that as "stuttering." He was bewildered. The children were doing certain behaviors in order to "help them get the words out," and those behaviors were called stuttering. When they did something else in order to not do those behaviors, people also were calling that stuttering too. Their only recourse, then, was to do something else so they wouldn't do what they just did. Does this sound confusing? It was confusing to the children too! Yet, one can observe the same behavior in adults. When was the last time that you did something similar, for example jerking your head backwards, so you would not tense your jaw and prolong a sound?

Children in their early teens often report more magical beliefs about stuttering than do the younger children. When some 12 or 13-year-olds were asked to discuss the question "What is stuttering like?" one 13-year-old boy reported that it is like trying to ride an untamed horse. He worried about when it (the "stuttering horse") would shy away from a word, would balk at the sight of a word or would begin to "buck" on a word. He felt that the only thing he could do was hang on as hard as he could, keep a tight rein on the horse and just "hope" that the horse wouldn't be too violent. Another 13-year-old reported that talking was like Indian wrestling. He constantly had to strain and to struggle so that his opponent (his stuttering) didn't get the best of him. As he talked, he tried to overpower it. The children talked as if they had to fight *against* their "stutter." Their "stuttering" was an adversary with a mind of its own, and in most instances, they were afraid that it was stronger than they were. With this viewpoint, then, it is quite natural for the child to feel that he has to tense, to struggle, and to use his muscles to fight the "stutter." It has been my observation that adults who stutter generally do the same thing, although they may not explain so vividly the reasons for doing it.

As adults, you probably have stuttered for many more years than the children just discussed. Whereas they still are actively trying to "explain" to themselves the reasons why they tense and struggle, you may have forgotten to ask "Why?" anymore. You no longer question the necessity or helpfulness of doing the tensing or head jerking or eye blinking that you do. You just accept it as part of what you, as a stutterer, *have to do* to talk. This is unfortunate because then you do not direct your attention toward observing, studying, and experimenting with what you can do in order to talk without the tensing and struggling. Yet, you *can* learn to talk easily and effortlessly.

There is nothing inside your body that will stop you from talking. You have the same speaking equipment as anyone else. You have the ability to talk normally. You are doing things to interfere with talking because you think they help. You tense the muscles of your chest, throat, mouth, etc., in an effort to try and fight the "stutter." Yet these are the same muscles that you need to use in order to talk. You can't do both at the same time because you only have one set of muscles. Therefore, it is extremely helpful to begin studying what normal speakers do as they talk. This is what you want to learn to do. Observe carefully the way they move their mouth, lips and jaws as they are talking. Then, sit and talk in a room by yourself, or read in unison with someone else and study the feeling of movement as you talk. There is a certain "just right tensing" that you do as you move your jaw and tongue and lips. Study it! This is what you want to do when you talk. Now begin to look at what you do to interfere with talking when you do what you refer to as your "stuttering." If you begin to hold your breath or tense your jaw, for example, you cannot move as easily as you must do to talk the way normal speakers do. In short, you need to develop a sharp sense of contrast between what you are doing that you call "stuttering" and what you do as you just talk easily. Use a mirror or a tape recorder to help you observe what you are doing. Above all, get a feeling deep in your muscles of the movements involved in easy talking. Then you can become much more alert to what you are *doing* (not what's "happening" to you) as you tense and interfere with talking.

After careful observation and practice of what you do as you talk easily and on-goingly, as opposed to interfering with talking by tensing, stopping, or speeding etc., enter a few speaking situations that are not so threatening that you cannot observe your behavior. It has been my experience that ordinarily the person observes that he gets scared, or he gets a "feeling" that he was going to stutter, and he tenses. What is this feeling? Work to be able to tolerate it so you can observe it carefully. Enter more speaking situations. Answer some questions. To what is the feeling similar? Does the feeling *alone* make you unable to talk? Or, do you tense when you begin to experience the feeling? When you start to talk do you pay attention to what you want to do (the movement you want to make) or are you attending to the "feeling" waiting for it to tell you whether you will be able to talk or not? Study the feeling. If you study it in various situations as you are talking you will become aware that it is a feeling that is in no way special from any other feeling of fear or embarrassment, etc. It is very normal. However, it is a feeling to which you have learned to react by tensing, or by speeding or slowing your rate. Essentially, you react to it by *doing* extra muscular activity than is necessary to do in order to talk. When you become aware that the struggling behavior you call stuttering is something that you are *doing* as you talk, and not something that magically "happens to you," you are in a very good position to begin to change what you are doing as you talk so that you can talk easier. Then, you can begin to talk by starting to move easily, being willing to experience the feelings that you may feel, but to continue moving easily. You can tolerate a few bobbles as you do this. Then, you can begin to see that there is a way out of this jungle. There is a reason to become optimistic because it is within your ability to do it. It's essentially a problem of learning to just "let yourself talk." You have learned to do too much. You do things to interfere. Learn by observing and experimenting that these things do not help. Talking is essentially easy ongoing movement of the jaw, tongue and lips, etc. Tensing unnecessarily only gets in your way. Your success in countering the excessive tensing as you talk will depend upon two factors. The first involves the thoroughness with which you come to understand that there is no "stuttering" to be *fought, avoided* or *controlled*, other than the tensing you, yourself, perform. Once you understand this as you talk, your own tensing becomes a signal for you to begin reacting constructively by immediately easing off on the tensing and attending to the easy on-goingness of talking.

The second involves practice. You must practice talking easily as you would practice typing or playing the piano easily and on-goingly even though you had a feeling in your stomach or chest that you might "goof" it at some point. Then, expand your speaking situations—and practice—until you can talk comfortably at any time you choose to speak.

This is the beginning of therapy for you. From now on, it is up to you!

Do-It-Yourself Kit For Stutterers

Harold B. Starbuck

Dear Sir or Madam: In reply to your letter of complaint about our Do-It-Yourself Kit for Stutterers, I apologize for not including the instructions. However, the kit was supposed to be empty! You don't need any gadgets to correct your stuttering. You already have all the tools and equipment you need. As long as you've got your body, complete with movable parts, you're set to begin. Don't ever forget that even though you went to the most knowledgeable expert in the country, the correction of stuttering is still a do-it-yourself project. Stuttering is your problem. You stutter in your own unique way. The expert can tell you what to do and how to do it, but you're the one who has to do it. You're the only person on earth who can correct your stuttering. Here are your instructions:

The first thing you must become is an honest stutterer. By that I mean you've got to stop trying to be fluent. You have to stop struggling with your feared words. Go ahead and stutter on them. Let your stuttering come out into the open. Hit the block head on and let it run its course. Start by stuttering aloud to yourself. Stutter on every word you say. Stutter two or three times on every word. Get used to it and notice that as you stutter freely you can eliminate all those retrials, avoidances, and half-hearted speech attempts. Practice on your family and friends. They won't mind and will be rooting for you. This is a tough step, but do it in every speaking situation until you are stuttering freely. Don't try to talk fluently without stuttering.

Now that you are able to stutter openly and without fear or shame, you can begin to answer the question, "How do I stutter?" You've got to examine and analyze the act of speaking to see what errors you're making. You must be making mistakes somewhere or you would be speaking fluently. What are you doing wrong that makes your speech come out as stuttering? Speech is, after all, just a stream of air we inhale, reverse, and push out our mouths while we shape and form it into speech sounds. One must realize that you can't have speech unless you have the air coming out your mouth. Examine your speech breathing. Are you inhaling a sufficient amount. After the air is in and you're ready to talk, are you reversing it smoothly and starting an outward flow, or are you holding it in your lungs? Are you blocking it off in your throat at the level of your vocal folds? (This happens on most vowel blocks.) Are you humping your tongue up in the back of your mouth and blocking it there, as on K and G? Is the tip of the tongue jammed against your gum ridge blocking the air on T and D? Have you jammed your lips together so no air can flow out on P and B? No air flow means no speech, and hard contacts between any two parts of the speech mechanism result in a blocked air stream. Now examine yourself a little more closely. Examine the muscular movements, stresses, and strains you use in producing those hard contacts. Examine the muscular tensions and pressures. Is it any wonder you stutter? Speech is an act of almost continuous movement, and when you stop that movement you're in a stuttering position. In order to say any speech sound, you have to move into position to say that sound, move through it, and then move out of it into position for the next sound. Find out what and where your blockages and stoppages are, and what muscular tension causes them.

Is there a solution? There is to every problem! What you've got to do now is to correct every problem or error you've analyzed. We call this the *Post-block Process of Correction.* Here's how it works:

Stutter on a word. When the word is completed, stop completely and analyze all of the errors you made while all the tensions and pressures are still fresh. Now, figure out a correction for each error. For example, suppose the air was blocked off in your throat on a vowel sound. The correction is an open throat. You will have to concentrate on the throat area so no muscular action jams the vocal folds closed. Concentrate on keeping them open the way they were when you inhaled. Reverse the air stream slowly, start the sound, and say it.

Suppose that the lip muscles had jammed the lips shut into a hard contact which allowed no air to pass. The correction would be a light contact or, better, no contact at all between the lips. Concentrate on controlling the lip muscles so that the lips just barely touch, or almost touch, and air is able to flow between them. An important aspect here is movement out of the sound, so you have to control the lip muscles in their movement out of the sound as well as into it. The air flow must be coordinated with the lip movement so that the sound is produced as the lips form the sound.

Figure out a correction for every error as in the above examples. When you have all the necessary corrections figured out, you are ready to try the word again. Exaggerate your corrections at first when you say the word, paying more attention to how the word feels rather than to how it sounds. The sounds may be slightly distorted and prolonged at first. That's good. The prolongation is the result of slow careful muscular movements as you move into, through and out of the sounds. The distortion is the result of light loose contacts. Feel the controlled air flow; feel the controlled muscle movements as you move fluently through the word with no stoppages.

Do a good job on the Post-block Process of Correction. This is where speech correction takes place. Don't just say the words over again fluently after you stutter. Say them carefully, concentrating on the feelings of muscular action as you coordinate the breath stream with the formation of sounds. Concentrate on the feelings of movement and fluency.

In the above step, we worked on the stuttering after it happened. Now we're going to move ahead a bit and work on it while it's happening. To do this you still have to stutter. While you are stuttering (which means you've got to keep the block going longer than the average), you must analyze what is happening incorrectly. When the errors are analyzed, you can start making corrections such as stopping a tremor, loosening a contact, and getting rid of tension until you are producing the stuttered sound in a stable, correct way. Then you can initiate movement out of the sound and complete the word. We call this step the *Block Process of Correction.* You go through the same process as you did in post-block corrections, only now you should be able to do it while you are stuttering. By now you should be able to recognize your errors almost instantly and know what corrections have to be made. Make the corrections, smooth out the sound, and complete the word. Practice this on any word you say. Stutter on purpose, get it under your control, and say the word.

You've gone through the Post-block and Block Processes of Correction. Now let's work on the stuttering even earlier. Let's work on it before it ever happens. This is the *Pre-Block Process of Correction.* When you come to a word you're going to stutter on—don't! Stop just before you start that word. Analyze how you would have stuttered on it had you said that word. Figure out the needed corrections and use them, saying the word just as you would a post-block correction. Feel the movements and fluency here too. With very little practice, you can eliminate the pause period and prepare for any feared word as you approach it. Take advantage here of your anticipation, expectancy, and fear of stuttering. An excellent way to work on this process is to select any word, feared or not, figure out how you would normally stutter on it, then figure out corrections, and apply the corrections when you get to the word.

You're now using *Predetermined Speech*. You are determining beforehand what movements you have to make, and how you have to make them, in order to say sounds and words fluently. You should be speaking fluently now, but don't fall into the trap of thinking you are a normal speaker. Normal speech for you is stuttering speech. Be proud of your abnormal predetermined fluent speech. Use it. Keep up your skills of controlling your muscle movements that produce speech. You have to eliminate your errors before, or while, they are happening. Once your speech is out beyond your lips, you can't pull it back and correct it. You must monitor your speech as you are producing it. Monitor your air flow, your muscle movements as you form sounds, and your movements through and out of sounds. Feel your fluency, and don't worry about the sound. That will take care of itself if you take care of the mechanism that is producing it.

Now you know why the kit was empty!

Putting It Together

Charles Van Riper

Now that you have read all of these suggestions you probably have some mixed feelings of confusion, helplessness and even disappointment. Perhaps you were hoping that at least one of these stuttering experts would have found a quick, easy, magical cure for your distressing disorder. Instead, it is quite evident that no such panacea exists and that, if you want relief from your miseries, you've got to earn that relief by making some real changes in the way you react to your stuttering and to your listeners and to yourself. As Dr. Emerick says, "The first thing to do is to admit to yourself that you need to change, that you really want to do something about your stuttering." Perhaps you are willing to make that admission but have some reservations about having to do what Dr. Boehmler calls the "dirty work of therapy." Some of the suggested procedures may at the moment seem far beyond your courage or capacities. Is the pay-off worth the cost?

All these authors answer that question with a resounding yes. I know these writers. They talk well and live well. All of them were severe stutterers. All of them know from personal experience your self doubts and the difficulties of self therapy but universally they insist that you need not continue to suffer, that you can change yourself as they have changed themselves and can become fluent enough to make the rest of your life a very useful and rewarding one. Perhaps you have already had some speech therapy and have failed and so feel that nothing can be done. If so, reread what Dr. Freund has told you about the success of his own self therapy after the best authorities in Europe had treated him unsuccessfully. Or you may be feeling that you are too old to begin now. If so, read what Dr. Sheehan had to say about the 78 year old retired bandmaster. Or you may be saying that you cannot do it alone without help, yet many of the authors agree with Dr. Starbuck's statement that essentially "The correction of stuttering is a do-it-yourself project. Stuttering is *your* problem. The expert can tell you what to do and how to do it, but you are the one who has to do it. You are the only person on earth who can correct your stuttering." While most of these writers would prefer to have you get competent professional guidance, they do not at all feel that it is impossible for you to get real relief without it. "Get help if you can," advises Professor Czuchna, "but if not, help yourself. You can!" They would not write so earnestly if they were not sure that you can do much to solve your difficulties. Moreover, you must remember that this is not the kind of false assurance or hope that you have received from others who never stuttered. This comes straight from persons who have known your despair and lack of confidence, from stutterers who have coped successfully with the same problems that trouble you.

At the same time, and as a measure of their honesty, they are realistic. They hold out little hope for what you have long dreamed of—the complete cure. Universally, they insist or imply that you can learn to live with your stuttering and to be pretty fluent anyway. This may be hard for you to accept—as it was hard for them too. The present writer has worked with a great many stutterers and has helped most of them to overcome their handicaps but only a few of the adult ones ever become completely free from the slightest trace of stuttering in all situations always. As Dr. Sheehan, the psychologist, advises, "Don't waste your time and frustrate yourself by trying to speak with perfect fluency. If you've come into adult life as a stutterer, the chances are that you'll always be a stutterer, in a sense. But you don't have to be the kind of stutterer that you are now—you can be a mild one without much handicap." We find this thought expressed by many of the authors. Dr. Neely says, "My own experience has been that nothing 'cures' an adult stutterer but one can effectively manage stuttering so that it ceases to be a significant problem throughout life". Dr. Murray writes, that he has known many adult stutterers who achieved a good recovery but not one who claimed to be completely free from disfluency. Dr. Barbara, the psychiatrist, insists that one of the major reasons for the persistence of stuttering is that the stutterer tries to speak too perfectly too often, that he has a "Demosthenes complex." Throughout this book, you have read many suggestions for the modification of your stuttering, for learning to stutter in ways that permit you to be reasonably fluent and free from emotional upheaval or social penalty. If these authors have one common message to you, it is this—you can change your abnormal reactions to the threat or the experience of stuttering and when you do so, most of your troubles in communicating will vanish. Is this bad? Is this not enough? As Dr. Emerick says, we cannot promise you a rose garden, but we can offer you a much better communicative life than the fearful, frustrating one you now endure.

But you may protest that you don't know where or how to begin. If you will read this book again, you will find author after author saying that the first thing to do is to study your stuttering and its associated feeling. In this, there is remarkable agreement. As Miss Rainey, the public school speech therapist, suggested to the young man she interviewed, you should get a mirror, and a tape recorder if possible, and start observing how you stutter, perhaps as you make a telephone call while alone, so that you can know how much of your avoidances and struggle is unnecessary and only complicates your difficulty. Dr. Johnson, Dr. Dean Williams and Dr. Dave Williams offer important sets of very challenging questions that you can ask yourself as you do this observing. Dr. Trotter advises you to count and time your blocks as you listen to yourself on the tape recorder and insists that "you will probably find that your blocks were not as long as you thought they were and that you actually stuttered about half as much as you expected you would." Other authors provide other ways that you can use to study your stuttering and feelings but all of them feel that this is how you should begin.

All of us know that this process of confronting yourself will not be pleasant but we also know you will find, as you observe and analyze what you do and feel when stuttering or expecting to stutter, that you will then know what you have to change. And will want to! Besides, isn't it about time you stopped pretending that you are a fluent speaker? Isn't it time, as Dr. Starbuck phrases it, for you "to become an honest stutterer," to come to grips with your problem, at least to look at it objectively?

To do so, you will have to accept another suggestion that these authors make almost unanimously. You've got to talk more and avoid less. You've got to start giving up what Miss Rainey called your "camouflage," the sort of tricks that Professor LaPorte lists for you in his article. We know that this too will be hard to do but over and over again you will find these writers insisting that they had to overcome their panicky need to hide their stuttering before they began to improve. They tell you, as Dr. Moses advises, to bring your stuttering into the open, to let it be seen and heard rather than concealed as though it were a dirty shameful thing rather than a problem that you are trying to solve. How can you possibly know what you have to change if you refuse to look at it? Aren't you tired to the bone of all this running away and hiding? Different authors outline different ways of decreasing this avoidance but you should be impressed by their basic agreement that you should admit, display and confront your stuttering openly and objectively.

There is another point on which almost all of them also agree. It is that you can learn to stutter much more easily than you now do and that when you master this, you will be able to speak very fluently even if you may continue to stutter occasionally. As Dr. Sheehan says, "You can stutter your way out of this problem." The idea—that it is unnecessary to struggle when you feel blocked and that there are better ways of coping with the experience—may seem very strange at first but if this book holds any secret for successful self therapy, it lies here. These writers say it in different ways. Dr. Aten advises you "to learn to substitute easy, slower, more relaxed movements for rushed, tight, forced movements," and to learn to decrease the tension. Dr. Trotter suggests that you "simplify" your stuttering. Dr. Emerick describes the process as getting rid of the excess baggage, the unnecessary gasps and contortions and recoils. In his account of his own self therapy, Dr. Gregory tells how he experimented with different ways of stuttering before he overcame his fear of it. Other authors tell you to learn to stutter slowly and easily. What they all seem to be saying is that it is possible to stutter in a fashion which will impair your fluency very little. Indeed, Dr. Murray suggests that if you study your stuttering, you will find that you already have some of these short, easy moments of stuttering in your speech and that if you will recognize them, they can serve as goals. If you read this article again, you will find him saying, "If you can learn to whittle the others down to similar proportions, most of your scoreable difficulty will have disappeared" and that "there are countless ways in which to stutter. You have a choice as to how you stutter even though you may not have a choice as to whether or not you'll stutter." Along with other authors, Dr. Agnello says that you should try different ways of stuttering, that you need not remain "bound" to your old patterns of stuttering. The present writer, now sixty-seven years old, agrees. For years he tried to keep from stuttering and only grew worse. Not until he found that it was possible to stutter easily and without struggling did he become fluent. He was born at the age of thirty years and has had a wonderful life ever since. How old are you?

So we suggest that you reread this book, this time to work out the design of your own self therapy. Your stuttering won't go away. There are no magical cures. You will not wake up some morning speaking fluently. You know in your heart that there is work to be done and that you must do it. This book contains many suggestions, and many guidelines. Your job is to sort out and organize those that seem appropriate to your own situation, to devise a plan of self therapy that fits your needs, and then begin the changing that must take place. Why spend the rest of your life in misery?

The Speech Foundation of America is a non-profit charitable organization dedicated to the prevention and treatment of stuttering. If you feel that this book has helped you, send a contribution to Speech Foundation of America, P. O. Box 11749, Memphis, Tennessee 38111. Contributions are tax deductible.